<u>Heal Thyself</u>

<u>Naturally</u>

Researched
Target Foods, Botanicals,
And Nutritionals

By

Jacquie Nelson Walburn
BS Nutrition
Gastrointestinal Mastery Certification
Condition Specific Nutrition and Lifestyle Coach
Empowering YOU to take back YOUR health

Designing Bio-Individual programs
using target dietary protocols, target foods,
botanicals, and nutritionals
@ RealHealthSolns.com

Copyright © 2014
Updated 2019

Dedicated to:

Jack Nelson
My father, who encouraged me to think for myself.

Starlyn Nelson
My sister, who helped put me on the path.

Betty Nelson
My grandmother, who never gave up on helping me
fixing my physical problems when the regular Western
medicine abandoned me.

Brad Nelson
My brother who asked me for help when his
neurodegeneration/Parkinson's began when doctors had
nothing & got his life back with my guidance.

Pharma vs. Natural

Facts: If a natural remedy is found, drug companies cannot patent it & make money. Many obstacles prevent new discoveries from reaching the public: Red tape, medical politics, Big Pharma, Big Ag, professional egos, turf wars, big money interests, etc.

As such, we are decades behind Europe & Asia. "In Germany, approximately 40% of all medical doctors prescribe homeopathic remedies or refer patients to practitioners who do," says Dr. Stengler. "Over 70,000 registered homeopaths practice in India. France – 6,000 physicians & 18,000 pharmacies sell homeopathic remedies. Britain has Royal London Homeopathic Hospital".

- ✓ **'Healthcare'** or 'Sick care' is big money based on acute care methodologies, **not chronic or preventative care**.

- ✓ **US is largest consumer** of Pharmaceuticals & has biggest lobbying group in the world

- ✓ **Pharmaceuticals only manage chronic conditions**

- ✓ 5% of hospital admissions are due to **negative drug reactions** (JAMA).

- ✓ **106,000 hospitalized patients die** each year from adverse reactions caused **by drugs** making adverse drug reactions the 4th leading killer (JAMA)

- ✓ **16,000 people die each year** in US alone from adverse reactions to **over-the-counter** (OTC) non-steroidal anti-inflammatory drugs (NSAIDs) per JAMA

- ✓ **Most pharmaceuticals are:** synthetic isolated chemicals designed to alter body chemistry at the cellular level & are not biocompatible, deplete nutrients, & cannot duplicate any substance found in nature as 'unpatentable' where botanicals contain dozens of compounds that usually work synergistically.

The **biggest problems** in recommending natural treatments, therapies, or cures are:

1. **AMA does not allow** doctors to prescribe natural remedies.
2. **So much information** that most doctors/people do not have the time to read through it all & keep up.
3. **They cannot be patented** & are not FDA regulated.
4. **Finding the potency** required to achieve test results. I have listed who/where to get "study" doses. I have also personally found not all supplements are created equal. Some have preservatives, some have fillers, some are x-rayed in the shipping process decreasing potency, and others may stress other systems in the body.
5. Just like some drugs, a 90% success rate still means it does not work for everyone.
6. Dr William Douglass says "big Pharma gets help from "medicrats" in CDC, EPA, & FDA with bribes disguised as research grants, consultation fees, & other forms of payola to help them develop a 'cure'."

<u>Key of abbreviations</u>

Bold	-	Name of herbal/homeopathic ingredient
"Bold"	-	Brand name formulated/used in study
↑	-	symbol for increase/improve
↓	-	symbol for reduced/decreased/lowered
dig	-	abbreviation for digestion
circ	-	abbreviation for circulation
chol	-	abbreviation for cholesterol
BP	-	abbreviation for blood pressure
Stims	-	abbreviation for stimulates
Inflam.	-	abbreviation for inflammation
Bact'l	-	abbreviation for bacterial
Prop's	-	abbreviation for properties
Fcn	-	abbreviation for function
Sol'n	-	abbreviation for solution

Disclaimer

Seen the drug commercials? Heard the side effects? Most pharmaceutical drugs treat symptoms only to manage symptoms. The underlying root cause is still there & will continue to cause problems in other parts of the body until addressed.

This information is a **summary** of research I found from reputable institutions, medical schools, journals, practitioners, & clinical studies/trials. It is provided for the reader to do their **own research,** discuss options with their doctor (regular, functional, integrative, or naturopathic), & decide what is best for them.

I believe every doctor and patient should be aware of all possible treatments available, so they can do what's in the best interest of the patient. Many natural solutions are less expensive than prescription medications making them a more affordable choice for some. I have not listed interactions here with other naturals or medications unless mentioned in the research.

This information is not presented to self-treat without a trained medical practitioner. Who you choose is entirely up to you. I have provided reference websites where you can locate practitioners if you so desire as they should be a member of your health care team. Some insurance companies will cover some alternative practices. No harm in asking.

I am also sure this is not a complete listing. There are many other natural alternatives out there but I chose to only list those that I had read the research, clinical studies, or trials mentioned.

The listings here do not reflect any preference or sponsorship on my part. They are basically listed in the order to which I found them. Some of my sources appear to be sponsored by nutritional research groups, boards, or distributors.

Resources & Info –

- American Association of Naturopathic Doctors-AANP (703-610-9037/ www.naturopathic.org)
- American Herbalist's Guild (AHG), www.americanherbalistsguild.com
- National Institute of Herbal Medicine (NIMH) www.nimh.org.uk/
- National Cert. Comm. of Acupuncture & Oriental Medicine (NCCAOM-www.nccaom.org),
- International Academy of Compounding Pharmacists (www.iacprx.org)
- Health Science Institute (www.HSIBaltimore.com)
- American College for Advancement in Medicine (www.acam.org) 800-532-3688
- International College of Integrative Medicine Directory (www.icimed.com)
- American Assoc. of Enviro. Medicine www.aaem.com.
- Herb-Drug Dangers on www.BottomLineSecrets.com/special
- BottomLine/Health – www.BottomLineSecretes.com
- Nat'l Ctr for Complementary & Alternative Medicine, nccam.nih.gov
- Institute for Cooperative Medicine/Better Health for better living. www.bhforbl.com/b_panel.html
- PubMed.com
- American Botanical Council, www.herbalgram.org
- **Dr. Jonathan V. Wright's** Nutrition & Healing (www.wrightnewsletter.com)
- **Dr. Mark Stengler**, MD Natural Healing.
- **Dr. Mercola, MD.** Mercola.com
- **MindBodyGreen.**com
- **Dr Tom O'Bryan** thedr.com
- **DrAxe.com**
- Dr Osborne glutenfreewarrior.com
- Dr Pompa Revelationhealth.com
- Greenmedinfo.com
- Izabelle Wentz PharmaD thyroidpharmacist.com
- **Other Leading researchers/practitioners =** Dr. Gary Null, PhD; Dr. Bruce West, MD; Dr. Richard Linchitz, MD; Dr. Robert J Rowen, MD; Dr. William V. Judy; Dr. John W Nelson, MD; Dr. David G. Williams; Dr. William Campbell Douglass II, MD; Dr Julian Whitaker, MD (**Whitaker Wellness Institute, Ca),** Dr Dennis Clark, Dr Susan Lark, MD; Dr Frank Shallenberger, MD, Dr Gooing, DC Costa Mesa, CA, JJ Virgin, Paleomom.com, Dr Mowll, Dr Terry Wahls

Table of contents

Healing Dietary Protocols: Pros and Cons

Dietary protocol is the first order of business for any illness/
condition/symptoms as it is directly linked to 'Food is Medicine',
'the terrain is everything' & 'all health and disease starts in the gut'.
That's Hippocrates 413 BC!

Research has now identified inflammation/stress as root cause to
all chronic conditions linking them to **autoimmunity** but we need
to connect the dots here. Anything coming into the body that causes
inflammation irritates the gut as to cause 'leaky gut' where intestinal
materials leak into the blood stream bringing an immune response that
then circulates these offending items and the inflammation they cause
all around the body that start the attack cycle on our own tissues.
There are now over 150 conditions linked to the **autoimmune
spectrum.** From weight gain, diabetes, arthritis to Hashimoto's,
dementia, Alzheimer's, & so on.

We are also living in the most toxic, contaminated, polluted world
humans have ever had to deal with and, quite frankly, the body is
struggling to keep up the detox schedule. Most chronic diseases are
linked to gut health (terrain), nutrient deficiencies, stress, toxicity, &
low-grade infections. Healing begins by ***making a decision*** to change.

We have all been betrayed by the 50 year failed 'Standard American
Diet' (SAD) food pyramid experiment focused on the over-
consumption of refined carb's and the low fat/industrial oils craze.

The new food pyramid has now been turned upside down!

Dietary Protocols for Healing Chronic Conditions:

Paleo (AKA: Caveman diet) – similar to 'Whole30'
  - ➢ **The goal**: Break the habit of living on processed junk food &
    beat sugar/carb addiction.
  - ➢ **Best for**: to see if food alone can reverse health conditions.
  - ➢ **Do's**: *Organic* proteins, *nutrient dense* vegetables, fruits, nuts, seeds.
  - ➢ **Don'ts**: all grains, dairy, alcohol, additives, sugars,..
  - ➢ **Difficulties**: Intense for 5-7 days to kick carb's/sugar. After
    that, easier as gut flora adjusts.
  - ➢ **Benefits**: Many see dramatic results in 30 days and break the
    habit of eating junk food - even healthy junk food (store Gluten-
    Free baked goods, sweetened yogurt, …).

AIP (auto-immune Paleo protocol)

➢ **The goal**: Eliminates common allergens, foods that damage the gut lining causing leaky gut, or feed bad microbes contributing to dysbiosis/SIBO – Paleo+ nightshades, many nuts/seeds, coffee, alcohol, sugar substitutes. Note: most common deficiencies - Vitamin D/B12, Zn/Omega 3's

➢ **Best for:** Those struggling with 'AI's not reversed with 'paleo' or gluten/dairy free diet (Dr Hyman – 88% do).

➢ **Do's**: Organic meats/fish, **8-12 Cups *nutrient dense* vegetables**, **1-2 C** fruit, herbs, sea salt. Eggs, nuts, and gluten-free grains/flours are reintroduced 1 by 1 in the reintroduction phase and allowed after if tolerated.

➢ **Don'ts - Not allowed foods** (to start):
   ✓ <u>Grains</u> – wheat (breads/pasta), rice, corn, barley, rye, pseudo grains (millet, amaranth, etc.)
   ✓ <u>Legumes</u> – all beans includes peanuts/beans/hummus, etc.
   ✓ <u>Dairy</u> – all sources of dairy, even raw or fermented (coconut yogurt/kefir OK)
   ✓ <u>Nuts/seeds</u> - all nuts/seeds (cashews/almonds/quinoa/sunflower/sesame/chocolate/coffee….)
   ✓ <u>Eggs</u> - especially the *white part of the egg*
   ✓ <u>*Nightshades*</u> - tomatoes, potatoes, peppers, eggplants, goji berries, and several spices
   ✓ <u>Industrial 'seed' oils</u> – Stick to unrefined olive (EVOO), coconut/MCT, and avocado oils
   ✓ <u>Processed/Preservative foods</u> - anything that comes out of a package or box (& avoid cans when possible).
   ✓ <u>Alcohol</u> - disrupts microbiome & induces leaky gut.
   ✓ <u>Sugar/starches/some fruits/yeasts</u> – Sweet, starchy, yeast-containing foods (even fermented) contribute to gut microbiome imbalances/dysbiosis as feeds the 'bad' gut microbes.

➢ **Temporary or permanent:** can be a life-long/lifestyle dietary modification for chronic AI conditions or temporary restriction with goal to reintroduce (regular paleo) foods after sensitivities are discovered, and autoimmune symptoms are reversed.

➢ **Difficulties:** Each phase lasts 3-6 months. Strict phase 1 then reintroduction phases.

➢ **Common struggles:** Cost is common misconception. Coconut oil & most veggies are inexpensive and can up calories without breaking the bank. Make sure eating enough calories/carb's, especially if already a healthy weight. Another struggle - too much alternative flours and maple syrup to re-create sweet treats & breads. Keep as occasional treats.

➢ **Benefits:** The elimination of problematic foods & an increase in vegetables to support the natural healing process to correct deficiencies/imbalances as provides building blocks the body needs to heal.

Ketogenic/Low Carb-High Fat (LCHF) Dairy optional

➢ **The goal:** To move body into ketosis, producing ketones, & running on *fat as fuel* rather than carb's.

➢ **Best for:** Weight loss as burns fat or for difficult to manage chronic health problems (diabetes,…).

➢ **Do's:** Eat fat, burn fat, get thin. Focuses on ketosis by limiting carb's (about 50 grams/day), upping fat (60%+ of Calories) so body runs on fat for energy - non-starchy vegetables, meat, high-fat oils/nuts/butters, avocadoes, fish, dairy or not. *¾ of every meal is nutrient dense veggies/6-10 Cups/day.*

➢ **Don'ts:** Focus is fat to carb ratio, so grains, rice, sugars/limited fruit, eat mostly berries ½ C – 1 C, & not too much protein.

➢ **Temporary or permanent:** For weight loss, yes. For chronic conditions, this is a *lifestyle* **change** advancing to carb cycling.

➢ **Difficulties:** Simple, but difficult. Transitioning into ketosis can make some feel sick for a few days as body adapts.

➢ **Common struggles:** To stay in ketosis, you can't really 'take a day off' or even enjoy a piece of cake without setting you back for weeks and having to adjust back into ketosis.

➢ **Benefits:** Stay under carb's/day, you can almost *eat all you want*. Easy transition to intermittent fasting. You run off fat so not hungry, improves gut health, overall health, & more energy, blood sugar, inflammation. ***Track on cronometer.com***

Vegan

➢ **The Goal**: reduce the burden on the environment of commercially processed/prepared animal product typically fed GMO grains (not natural food source) and the damage it causes to the body – hormones, antibiotics,…...

➢ **Do's**: organic plant foods - fruits, vegetables (including roots), fermented foods (sauerkraut, kimchi,…) along with 100%

organic whole grains (wheat, oats, quinoa, rice), legumes, nuts/butters/milks, seeds, seaweed, ***organic*** fermented soy,....

➤ **Don'ts:** all animal products – eggs, milk, meat, fish, gelatins, processed/packaged foods, can choose to avoid gluten as well.
➤ **Difficulties:** Staying organic, non-GMO, dairy free.
➤ **Common Struggles:**
  ✓ Getting ***enough protein*** to maintain muscle & development (pea protein/hemp powder, nuts/seeds, quinoa can help)
  ✓ Other ***nutrient deficiencies*** that tend to be higher among vegans (B_{12}, zinc, calcium absorption, omega 3s – algal forms avaiable), especially those consuming processed foods.
  ✓ Higher intake of ***antinutrients*** - phytic acid/lectins, high carbs can be problematic
➤ **Benefits:** weight management, heart health, reduced risk for metabolic syndrome, high antioxidant intake, improved gut health (prebiotics, fiber). *When done correctly*, can be healthy for some.

What do they all have in common:

1. All improve weight & health - Alzheimer's, diabetes, arthritis, heart,…
2. No processed/packaged foods or industrial oils
3. No alcohol, No (or limited) gluten/dairy
4. All organic, high veggies, fermented foods
5. Supplement B12, D, K, magnesium, zinc, Omega 3's, probiotics

Other diets are just tweaking for personal health status – low FODMAPS, oxalates, salicylates, histamine, elimination, elemental, SDC, GAPS, body ecology, PAMM (Mediterranean), …....

The bottom line: most do better to transition slowly & monitor how you feel as you make changes to your diet. Focus on factors - energy levels, well-being, sleep, skin, digestion.

If you need help, I can design a program for you at RealhealthSolns.com

Multi-symptomatic– claim to do many things/do it all
(prolong life/eliminate multitude of problems)

➢ **Indium** – mineral; research shows better uptake of all minerals = improves digestion/circulation/brain fcns/liver/heart/ lungs/kidneys/adrenals/pituitary/thyroid + help w/osteo-porosis/weight/diabetes/BP/cholesterol. East Park Research, Inc. www.eastparkresearch.com. (Several sources)

➢ **Vinpocetine** – prescription in Europe = ↑ short-term memory (40%), relieves - Alzheimer's/Parkinson's/dementia/de-pression (76% of cases), elim. headaches (78%), eye-sight ↑ (70%), ↓ inner ear problems (tinnitus/vertigo in 70%), insomnia (78%), prevent/ treat strokes. (Several sources)

➢ **HGH – *"Symbiotropin Pro-HGH"*** – stims release from pituitary - IGF-1 level increased 30% - ↓ body fat/cholesterol/ ↑ vision/memory/energy/hair growth/skin. Ctr for Nat'l Med. Dispensary www.cnm-inc.com. Or *"**Red Deer Antler Velvet**"* – ↑ muscle strength/inflam./nerve impulses/athletic performance/ wound healing/regulate BP/treat arthritis/↓ body fat/antiviral/ tumor properties. Lifestar Millennium, Inc (HSI). **Arginine/ ornithine/glutamine** – 3 AAs that stim's *HGH* production.

➢ **Ubiquinone** – converted CoQ_{10}-enzyme decreases w/age = deteri-oration tied to heart/baldness/wrinkles/eyesight/ hearing/arthritis/ age spots/bladder control/prostate. Noble prize Dr Mitchell/Judy, AMA/JIM/JN/ US Gov NIH/UCLA Med Schl/IN U Med School.

➢ **Glutathione (GSH)** – disease-fighting, immunity-boosting, antioxidant, energy-producing, detoxifier, enzyme activator/ regulator, feeds the brain, protects liver. 1000s of books… liposomal encapsulation.

➢ **Jiaogulan** –inhibits tumor growth/normalizes BP/free radical damage/immune system/sleep/cholesterol. Tea or caps. Prev = 1 cap/day, treat = 1 cap 3/day (HSI)

➢ **Vit D** – now linked to 2,000 genes & 20+ organs. Low levels linked to immunity/depression/asthma/cancer/ Alzheimer's/ dementia/flu/tooth decay. Recommendations now between 2,000 – 10,000 IU/day. (Mercola + many others)

➢ **Arjuna** – well documented for ↓ LDL/over-all cholesterol + angina attacks w/o side effects (out performed ISMN) + ↓ systolic BP, ↓ BMI (wt loss), corrects atherosclerosis, fight several cancers, l types of E. coli, & Salmonella infections. "***Arjuna – Cardiac Tonic***" (Himalaya USA 800-869-4640)

➢ **Resveratrol** –*Moravian* red wine ext.= *French Paradox*; anti-aging, ↓ blood clots/bad chol/plaque dep./balance hormones/anti-inflam/macular degeneration/COX-2 inhibitor/rejuvenates/immunity/correct existing conditions/diseases. Harvard/Boston/ Yale/No Western.." ***Vinotol"*** –BioNutrients, Inc. 800-619-6987; "***Botanical Vitality"*** Great Life Labs 800-695-5995; "***Revatrol"*** Renaissance Hlth 866-482-6678 (several)

➢ **Beta-glucan** – origin aqua-culture/mushrooms. Based on idea that most ailments = microinfections. Boosts immunity, treats many chronic ailments (arthritis/chronic fatigue/cancer/HIV/herpes/cold/flu/allergies/parasitic/bact'l infections). "***Immutol"*** Immuno-corp . www.immunocorp.com

➢ **Pregnenolone** - ↑ energy/mood/immunity, ↓ rheumatoid/osteoarthritis/chronic joint & muscle pain/insomnia/cardio/LDL/thyroid conversion of T4 to T3, cortisol/stress, & hormonal balances of DHEA, progesterone, estrogen, & testosterone. Silver Edge Hlth/Nut 800-528-0559. (several sources)

➢ "***StemEnhance"*** – from dark greens/algae. Research showing stimulates release of own stem cells from bone marrow, to blood stream, seek out damaged cells & replace them. www.E3Live.com/888-800-7070. (HSI)

➢ **Di-indole methane (DIM)** – a plant nutrient in cruciferous veggies that balances hormones/prevents estrogen dominance (menopausal/prostate problems)/ fights depression/anxiety/fatigue/hair loss/thyroid problems/reduces risk for abnormal cell growth. (per quotes from Jl of Endocrine & Metabolism/Jl of Bio Chem/Br Jl of Cancer/Jl of Clinical Endocrinology)

➢ **"*Pain & Brain Rescue formula*"** –curcuminoids from **turmeric** + **Boswellia** (anti-inflam.) - relieves arthritis/ neutralizes metabolic wastes + **Gugulipid** converts excess cholesterol/burns stored fat/ ↑ levels of prostacyclin - zap abnormal platelets/inner cleansing of all major organs/↑ immunity/anti-bacterial/viral/fungal, ↓ stress/fatigue, **Bioerine** to absorb/use nutrients/better skin & energy. Institute for Vibrant Living 800-218-1379

➢ **Procaine** – "*GH-3/H-3 Plus*" repairs damaged cell membranes to improve nutrient uptake by 70%, ↓ % get diseases, ↓ infections – help w/acne/arthritis/depression emphysema/ cholesterol/heart disease/Hodgkin's/migraines/MS/osteoporosis/Parkinson's. Covered on 60 mins – 100 mil. people use. "*Ultra H-3*" 1-2 x/day. www.unikeyhealth.com. (many sources)

➢ **Sepia** – made from ink of cuttlefish. Treats hormone-related conditions = PMS/menopause/irregular menstrual cycles/ ovarian cysts/fibrocystic breast syn./ hormonal headaches/ bladder infections/ hypo-thyroid/low libido/migraines/prostate enlargement/psoriasis/sinusitis/incontinence during menopause/uterine prolapse/vaginitis/varicose veins. (Stengler)

➢ **Turmeric/curcumin** – most studied nutrient - research demonstrates useful for ↓ breast/lung/prostate/colon cancer (anti-metastasis/causes apoptosis/protective/prevents angiogenesis + treat breast cancer/IBS/Crohn's/Alzheimer's/ Ulcers/colitis/diabetes/ PMS/arthritis/ maybe cystic fibrosis. Considered a potent anti-inflammatory, powerful anti-oxidant, reduces free radicals. (many sources)

➢ **Astaxanthin** – from H. pluvialis microalgae – prevents oxidation/mutation of cells & ARMD/anti-inflammatory/ decrease LDL/cancer risks/heart disease/cholesterol/neurodegenerative diseases. AstaFactor Mera Pharm., Inc. 800-480-6515 www.astafactor.com. (several sources)

➢ **Omega-3 oils** (fish/calamarie/algal/flax seed oils) 1 T 2x/day = decreases cholesterol/heart disease/rheum. arthritis/ joint pain/breast cancer/asthma/diabetes/insulin resistance/ menstrual cramps/PMS/psoriasis/ eczema/stroke/flaky skin/ split-brittle nails/ "bumpies" on back of arms. (several sources)

➢ **Goji/Ningxia Wolfberry** – use 100+ yrs in China/ Japan/ Tibet. Potent antioxidant w/zeanthin & carotenoids = increase WBC/hemoglobin/eyes/liver/ kidneys/immune-globulin A/circulation/decrease tumor growth/cataracts/ LDL/ plaque/BP/fat comp/blood sugar. "*OCS-147*" combines w/selenium (flush toxins) + turmeric (inflam.) + B complex (homocysteine) BioNutrigenics, Inc800-863-8138

➢ **SAMe** (butanedisulfonate form enteric coating) – 400 - 1200 mg/day treats depression by contributing to pro-duction of dopamine/serotonin + arthritis/muscle pain/ low energy characterized in fibromyalgia/chronic fatigue syndrome & maintain glutathione (antiox). (sev sources)

➢ **Apple-cider Vinegar** – decreases cholesterol/BP/plaque from arteries/balances pH/increases heart function + circulation/ strengthens arteries/veins/less pain/controls appetite/weight loss/kills inf./↓ varicose veins/digestive aid/bloating/acid reflux. Many sources.

➢ **Seabuckthorn** – seed oil caps./juice/creams/teas. Treats burns/grafts/infections/gastric ulcers/decreases inflammation/ support liver/retard growth of tumors/anti-bact'l/skin aging. Kettle Valley www.kvsbt.com (HSI)

➢ **Boswellia** serrata extract (frankincense) - compare to NSAID pain relievers/lowering inflammation/reducing joint/arthritis pain/helping fight cancer/speeding up healing infections/may preventing autoimmune diseases, rebuild cartilage.

➢ **Dimethylglycine** (DMG) – works on cellular level to restore virtually all bodily function by enhancing healing effects of other nutrients/restores oxygenation levels to cells, tissues, organs to fight infections/decreases homo-cysteine/ cholesterol/triglycerides/angina & enhance immunity/cellular detox/liver/physical endurance & performance. (Balch/Sahelian/Kendall) TheSilverEdge.com

Acne – 1st step -limit/eliminate IGF1 insulin-producing carb's – grains/fruit. Also linked to gut imbalance (see healing diets)

➢ **Zinc** – acne associated w/DHT as high levels linked. Zinc reduces conversion & promotes healing. Also for burns/ colds. 45 mg/day. (Dr Stengler) **Zinc** – 50-60 mg + 2-4 mg **copper** + 1 T **flaxseed oil/**day. Boys, add 200-500 mcg **selenium**. Topical **4% niacin-amide** + 10% **Vit C** cream. Also = **pantothenic acid, cat's claw** for cystic acne.

➢ **Burdock** – eczema, acne, psoriasis, etc. Detoxifier = supports liver, destroys blood impurities (bacteria/ yeast), lymphatic drainage; improves digestion & elimination. It is rich in minerals, phytonutrients, & stimulates metabolism/healing. (Dr Stengler)

➢ **SSKI** – super saturated potassium iodide; pimples/ hang-nails/ cold sores/toenail fungus. *"Tri-Quench"* (50 SSKI/50 DMSO mix (**DMSO** = rub-on liquid avail. @ some HF Store or on-line that carries substances into the body through skin). It ↓ inflammation/scar tissue (Whitaker)

➢ **Tea tree oil** (Melaleuca alternifora oil) = anti-inflammatory/ analgesic/antiseptic/anti-bacterial/fungal/viral for **acne/** athlete's foot/boils/burns/cold sores/dandruff/insect bites/rashes/lice/warts/gingivitis (gargle). In a 5% extract cream or gel; as a soap; or 10 drops in 1 t water (not undiluted). Not for infants. (Stengler)

➢ **Black cumin seed oil** – mix with carrier oils like jojoba or coconut,….

ADD/ADHD – no more Ritalin® – addictive. Most naturopaths recommend do dietary changes 1st + DHA/GLA oil balances, probiotics, + no food colorings/preservative/dyes.

➢ **Do it w/diet** –1st, eliminating food allergies/sensitivities = elimination diets – Keto/AIP/Paleo (**see 'healing diets'** - no wheat/nuts/sugar/milk/soy…)/blood/muscle tests/radionics. Good multi-vit/mins + 50 mg Vit B_6 & 100 mg Mag. 6+ mos. (Dr Wright) + Check iron - low level may be link. (Dr Inglis)

- ➢ **EAT GOOD FATS: Omega 3 & 6 FA** (Dr Stengler+)
  - ✓ **Marine oils (algal/calamarine)** = 475 mg EPA, 151 mg of DHA + other omega 3 fatty acids or **Cod liver oil** = 300 mg GLA + 200 IU Vit. E mixed as tocopherols. Eliminate sugar/refined carbs/processed foods
  - ✓ **+ Evening primrose oil** = omega-6 EFA/GLA - 54 mg of GLA (750 mg of oil) + omega-3 oil supplement taken w/meals.
  - ✓ **+ Lycopodium clavatum** – homeopathic for mood & concentration
  - ✓ **+ phosphatidylserine** – (PS)– clinical trials w/over 90% w/dramatic improvement. Normal brain cell membrane function nutrient in fish/green veggies. (Balch/Stengler)

- ➢ **Inositol** - is used for diabetic nerve pain, panic disorder, high cholesterol, insomnia, cancer, depression, schizophrenia, Alzheimer's, **ADHD**, autism, promoting hair growth, psoriasis

- ➢ **Zinc** – common deficiency linked to brain health

- ➢ **Turmeric/curcumin** – inflammation, detoxing, support gut

- ➢ **Gotu Kola** – ↓ agitation/anxiety/insomnia/epilepsy/ **hyperactivity** (too much = rash + sedate)

- ➢ **Sulfur** – homeopathic. Cellular detox energy back **+ ADD**, detox's digestive tract. Def symptoms = always warm, sweats easily, no blankets, thirsty, likes sweet/spicy foods. 2 - 6C potency tabs 2/day for 2 wks. Skin may flare (detox). Stengler

- ➢ **Adaptogens** – ginkgo biloba, ginseng, ashwaganda. (calming)

- ➢ **GABA** – a neurotransmitter produced normally by the gut microbiome. Taking a GABA supplement, alone or in conjunction with traditional treatments, may help lessen symptoms of ADD and ADHD naturally. 250-400 mg 3x/day. DrAxe.com

Alcohol Use/Abuse

– Kills microbiome, stimulates release of dopamine followed by endorphins = happy & relaxed as boosts blood sugar, raises energy. But it's a depressant so next, leads to irritability & impaired function. In moderation (1/day), it can protect against diseases. Excessive over time increases risks for brain swelling/dementia/liver failure/heart disease/stroke/cancer/bone fractures/erectile dysfunction. Many heavy drinkers have hypoglycemia = cravings. Get tested. (Stengler)

➤ **Amino acids** – reduce cravings/withdrawal symptoms. **L-tyosine** 900 mg + **L-tryptophan** 400 mg + **L-glutamine** 2,000-3,000 mg (in divided doses) + **DLPA** 1,500 mg (in 3 divided doses – careful if hi BP/insomnia/anxiety/bipolar w/Dr help (not w/anti-depressants, no pheylketonuria)

➤ **Kudzu** – extract; a fast-growing vine. Harvard study found plant's flavones seem to turn off desire to drink. (Prev)

➤ **B Vits** – boost neurotransmitter production & fix deficiencies common to heavy drinkers. B Vit complex 50 mg + B-3/niacin no-flush 500 mg. (Dr Stengler)

➤ **Chromium** – helps balance blood sugar reducing urge. 200 mcg 2x/day (Dr Stengler)

➤ **Probiotics** – gut imbalance increases craving as bad bacteria flourish & good get killed off. Taking daily good bacteria replaces & cravings diminish.

➤ **L-Glutamine** – cuts cravings, heals gut lining. Dr Hyla Cass

Allergies

Am. Academy for Enviro. Medicine (aaem.com) = best single resource. Long-term use of steroids for asthma can cause liver/kidney damage. **Eliminate food allergies/sensitivities = see 'healing diets'**/skin tests/blood tests/muscle tests/electro-dermal tests/& radionics. Good multi + extra 50 mg Vit B_6 /100-400 mg Mag. 6+ months (Dr J Wright). ALCAT test can identify & tell you what & how to eliminate these causes. Chronic inflam = underlying root to allergies/asthma/arthritis/psoriasis/heart disease/cancer = IL-6 test. (Dr Stengler). Can also be linked to candida overgrowth.

➤ **Hives** – red clover tea 3-4 cps/day helps red/swollen skin

- ➤ *"Oralmat"* – Secale cereale extract liquid decreases/eliminate need for drugs – allergies/colds/flu/sinus/asthma. 3 drops under tongue per day. (HSI)

- ➤ **Urtica dioica** (stinging needles) 300 mg + **Quercetin** modulates immune system/heals leaky gut 1,000 mg 3-4/day - hay fever/sinuses/inflammation/sneezing/coughing (several).

- ➤ **D-Hist** – 40 million Americans use - treats root of cause w/**quercetin/stinging nettles/bromelain/NAC.** For many, no more drugs/inhalers necessary w/daily dose.

- ➤ **Sodium bicarbonate** (baking soda) 1-2 tsp into 6-12 oz of H_2O - drink rapidly for attacks. "**Trisalts** & **Alkala**" = more eff. Some Dr's prefer **sodium ascorbate**. (several)

- ➤ *"TaurImmune"* – Taurox/COBAT spray = combo of AA beta-alanine + taurine decreases symptoms by suppressing histamine release. Can add to meds. May have detox rxn. No transplants/immune def/pregnant. Biocentric Hlth 877-880-7800 www.biocentrichealth.com (HSI)

- ➤ **Nettle leaf + Quercetin** = herbal anti-histamines no drowsy. NL = 600 mg 3x/day + Q = 1,000 mg 3x/day (Dr Stengler)

- ➤ **Mullein** – herbal for coughs, chest congestion, mucus expectorate, anti-inflammatory effects on resp tract. 30-40 drops 3-4x/day (Dr Stengler)

- ➤ **Butterbur** – used in Europe to block pollen allergic symptoms (Dr Ronald Hoffman)

- ➤ **Beta-glucan** – Mushroom ext. Based on idea that most ailments = micro-infections. Boosts immunity, many chronic, long-term ailments cured – cold/ flu/**allergies**. "*Immutol*" Immunocorp www.immunocorp.com (several)

- ➤ **N-acetyl cysteine** (NAC) – amino acid derivative that boosts immune fcn/mucus-thinning prop's to help relieve wet cough w/phlegm/sinus congestion. 500-600 mg 3x/day (Stengler)

- ➤ **Berberine** – anti-histamine/immune modulator,….

- ➤ **Black Cumin seed oil** – reduces allergies & asthma when consumed (MGB).

Allergies, cont.

➤ **Bromelain** – enzyme from pineapples aids in protein dig. (IBS), thins blood, breaks down clots/plaques, angina, anti-inflam. (arthritis), & **mucus thinning agent (CF or sinusitis)**, improves surgery recovery time. 2,000 MCU/1,000 mg or 1,200 GDU/ 1,000 mg split into 500 mg 3x/day. (Dr Stengler) 1000 mg + 1 t baking soda in 1 cup H_2O (Dr Whitaker)

➤ **Tea tree oil** (Melaleuca alternifora oil) = anti-inflam/anti-septic/bacterial/fungal/viral for acne/ athlete's foot/boils/ burns/cold sores/ cuts/insect bites/**rashes**/lice/warts/ gingivitis (gargle). In a 5% extract cream or gel; as a soap; or 10 drops-1 t in water (not undiluted). Not infants. (Stengler)

Alzheimer's/Dementia/Memory – start with

prevention - avoid fluoridated water/aluminum – aspirin/baking powder/cans/anti-perspirants/deodorants/cheese/pesticides/tooth-pastes. Also called Diabetes III linked to blood sugar (90+)/insulin resistance (see 'healing diets').

➤ **ALA** – Alpha lipoic acid (fatty acid) in 1 study was given daily & it stabilized cognitive fcn. (Mercola)

➤ **Candida infection -** can be major player as linked to sugar & floods body w/toxins that cross blood-brain barrier. Clinical data = most test + for candida. (see candida) – Dr Teitelbaum

➤ **Memantine** – approved in Europe; protects brain from damage caused by glutamate = same effect as prescription **lithium**. Inhibits beta-amyloid secretions & helps chelate Al. Test lithium blood levels/thyroid function test. Add 1-2 T of **flaxseed oil** + 400IU **Vit E** daily + limit Al. (see hearing) + low-doses lithium aspartate or orotate shows in studies to block 6 major pathways. (Dr Wright)

➤ **B12 deficiency** – mimics problems. Take methyl-cobalamin best as sublingual, patch.

➤ **Rosemary** – essential oil improves acetylcholine in the brain

➤ **L-Glutamine** – fuel for immune cells, heal leaky gut/leaky brain linked to condition. Dr Osborne

➢ **Huperzine A** (HupA) – raises acetylcholine levels like drugs + protects brain from free radical damage. Significant improvements in cognitive/intellectual performance for **Alzheimer's**. In a study testing head-to-head w/drugs, out-performed them. China prescription for **dementia** (Stengler/HSI)

➢ **Galantamine** – ext from snowdrop flower blocks action of cholinesterase w/clinical trials surpassing prescription drugs by stopping progression & rejuvenating cognitive fcn. FDA approval pending. 24 mg/day for 3 –6 mos. **"Reminyl"** (HSI)

➢ **Ginkgo Biloba** – terpene lactones - bioflavonoids/anti-oxidants prevent/treat Alzheimer's (apprvd by German Gov. effective delay of mental deterioration) as it ↑ circulation to brain, + strokes/protects blood vessels/decreases inflam. 120-360 mg/day. Careful w/Coumadin/aspirin. (Stengler)

➢ **Zinc** – reduces conversion/promotes healing - Alzheimer's/ macular degeneration/…45 mg/day (Dr Stengler)

➢ **Hericium erinaceus/hedgehog fungus** – Asian remedy for **dementia**. **"Super Lion's Mane"** combo w/Maitake/Reishi + clinically tested to improve neurological fcn. (HSI)

➢ **Lion's Mane** – Stim's NGF/regenerates nerves/reduces plaque. GreenMedInfo

➢ **Iodine def** – leading cause of brain failure (WHO) or **normal pressure hydrocephalus** – fluid build up. (Williams)

➢ **Phosphatidyl serine** (PS) – 63 clinic trials/2,800 re-search papers – memory retention/word assoc. (Jl of Natural Med)

➢ **Inositol** - used for diabetic nerve pain, panic disorder, high cholesterol, insomnia, cancer, depression, **Alzheimer's**, ADHD, autism, promoting hair growth, psoriasis, & treating side effects of medical treatments with **lithium.**

➢ **Bacopa monnieri** – 14 separate studies - ↑ memory, reasoning skills, & learning. (Jl of Nat'l Med- Dr Bowen)

➢ **Niacin/Nicotinic acid deficiency:** No flush – raises acetylcholine. Those w/highest levels = 80% less likely to get Alz's. (Williams) & possible reversal. (Dr Andrew Saul)

HSI simple stuff:
- ➢ **DMAE** – helps brain halves communicate = verbal/creative
- ➢ **Lecithin** – can support short-term memory for all. (HSI)
- ➢ **GABA** – protects neural pathway overload/judgment
- ➢ **Omega 3's** – DHA/EPA brain's optimization/preferred food

- ➢ **Vit C/E** supp.- large doses prev/↓ incidence by 60%; slows prog. '02 study (JAMA); ↓ risk 70% over 4 yr per 2,000 IU/day.

- ➢ **PQQ** – for mitochondria regeneration in the brain, protective. Studies show significantly improves mental processing, works with CoQ10 for even better results.

- ➢ See multi-symptomatic:
  Vinpocetine/Curcumin/Turmeric/Vit D + Vit K

Arthritis – address diet – see dietary

(Many of these out performed Vioxx®, Remicade®, Celebrex®, Indo-merhacian® w/o side effects – ulcers, internal bleeding, liver/kidney damage+ may accelerate cartilage degeneration). **Warning**: prolonged use of **MSM** (1+ yrs) needs 50 mcg molybdenum supp. **Glucosamine** – can mess with blood sugar. **Chondrotin** – usually from shellfish (allergies). *Arthritis can be caused by too much Ca/too little Mg* = need 2 Ca: 1Mg (1000 Ca/ 500 Mg). **Chronic inflammation/heavy metals** = underlying root cause arthritis/psoriasis/diabetes/heart dis/cancer = IL-6 test.

- ➢ **Cetylmyrestoleate** (CMO) –eliminate symptoms (even severe) after 30-day course (93% partial - total remission). All nat'l veg. ext. Dr Harry W. Diehl @ Nat'l Inst. Of Hlth in MD. Study in Jl. of Pharma. Sciences. Silver Edge Hlt/Nut. 800-528-0559

- ➢ *"Flexagene"* – ↓ aches/swelling/repairs joints w/**Vincara** (Uncaria guianensis extract) turns down inflam. (Med Jl *Inflam. Research*) + **RNI 249** (Lepidium Meyenii ext.) stim's/rebuilds joints/turns on gene responsible for producing IGF-1 (insulin-like growth factor 1) helps build lean muscle, burn fat stores, maintains skin, normalizes blood sugar. Swiss Labs 800-619-7281

- ➢ **Bromelain** – enzyme from pineapples = ↓ inflammation. 500 mg 3x/day of std 2,000 MCU/1,000 mg. (Stengler) +**proteolytic enzymes** – breaks up fibrin scare tissues.

11

➤ *"TheraFlex"* = **Boswellia**/Ashwagandha/Shatavari for pain; Bromelain/**turmeric**/cinnamon for inflam.; ginger/licorice/ zinc/ astaxanthin/rehmannia/copper for detox/free radical eliminators; & **Bioperine** ext. (black pepper) ↑ bioavailability.

➤ **"Pain & Brain Rescue formula"** – curcuminoids from **turmeric** + **Boswellia** (anti-inflam.) relieves arthritis, neutralizes metabolic wastes, **Gugulipid** converts excess cholesterol, burns stored fat, ↑ levels of prostacyclin to kill abnormal platelets/inner cleansing of all major organs/ immune enhancer/anti-bacterial/viral/fungal/↓ stress/ fatigue, **Bioerine** to absorb/use nutrients in food, better skin, & energy. Institute for Vibrant Living 800-218-1379

➤ *"Pain Erase"* - all natural liquid developed under Dr. John W Nelson, MD that "closes the gates of pain" left open even after healing has occurred. Erases arthritis/knee/migraines/back/ neuropathy/bursitis/hip/tendonitis/sciatica/neck pain for hrs/days/weeks/even years. Harbor Hlth 888-859-9800

➤ **OPC** – 200 mg high quality **red grape seed ext**. made from whole red grapes (skin/stem/etc) rebuilds/↓ inflam./↑ flex/ recovery/pain/↑ immune. Dr. Halvorson, MD. *"OlyJoint Ultimate OPC"* + anthocyanidins (anti-oxid) 800-642-1571

➤ *"Nexrutine"* - Phellodendron's yellow bark – **berberine** to make super aspirin (huang-po) w/o side effects - study shows relief of pain/inflammation/ stiffness w/in 7 days. (Solanova)

➤ *"Triple Jointed"* – avocado soy unsaponifiables (ASU)/ undenatured type II chicken collagen (UC-II) & ginger boosts/restores aggrecan prod./slow & repairs osteoarthritis cartilage damage/decreases inflammatory factors/inhibits cartilage degradation. May help *Rheumatoid.* Baseline Nut'l

➤ **DMSO/MSM** – **DMSO** = liquid rubbed on w/cotton ball towards heart. Has been around for yrs but recently approved by FDA for humans – quick inflam./stiffness/ pain relief. **MSM** = caps/cream 2,000 mg/day + needs extra B Vit's. Can buy either straight or in *"Soothanol X2"* NorthStar Nut = DMSO +Emu oil+**MSM**+ Arnica+... relief + rebuild. 800-311-1950

➤ **Serratiopeptidase** (SP) ***"Arthro Enzyme"*** – from silk moths = blocks pain by stopping release of pain-causing Amines from inflamed tissues, drains harmful fluids, shrinking swelling, & speeds tissue repair, cleans up metabolic wastes, dissolves dead/damaged tissue, diabetic neuropathy. Used in Europe for 23+ years. Jl of Internal Med - 40 clinical studies.

➤ **Powerful Combo – Safe to take all 3** (White/Stengler)
  ✓ **Boswellia/Frankincense** = similar to glucosamine = ↓ inflam/pain/swelling, ↑ lubrication/flex/↑ repair/rebuild by 90% in 2 wks. 1,200 – 1,500 mg ext 2-3/day (65% std)
  ✓ **Willow bark extract.** – "natural" aspirin (synthetic's origin) w/o side effects/more effective.
  ✓ **Devil's claw** – So African plant - similar to ibuprofen/ cortisone - outperformed Vioxx® (not if ulcers/preg./ Coumadin) 1200-2500 mg/day aqueous ext. (powdered = 5-10 g/day) for pain/muscles.

➤ **Glucosamine** <u>Sulfate</u> **(not HCl)/MSM/Chondroitin** – (see heading warnings) only works for 50% due to B Vit. deficiency (add B's) = double blind studies for **osteo** ↓ inflammation, ↑ lubrication, & ↑ repair/rebuild. ***"Flexanol"*** (NorthStar) contains all 3 + **Boswellia**, EPA/DHA (omega-3 FA's), borage oil, + **shellfish free**. 800-311-1950. If can't take – try **Shark Cartilage** – same affects naturally. (several sources)

➤ **Infopeptides** – in colostrum. Regulates immune system – **rheumatoid** + **osteoarthritis** ***"Cytolog"*** (Natural Health Consultants)" 888-852-4993.

➤ **Hyaluronic Acid** (HA) deficiency – rooster comb ext; called "Cartilage in a bottle" stops breakdown of joint collagen from enzyme hyaluronidase that attacks HA = lubricates/decreases pain/inflammation/protects synovial fluid/repairs/restores joint collagen/dehydration. 9000 reports. Williams = boil "bone broth + egg shells". ***"Alliviate"*** = HA + Boswellia, ginger, white willow extract, Vit C. Inst for Vibrant Living 800-218-1379 (Stengler)

➤ **Niacinamide** – no-flush 1000 mg 3x/day for 3-4 weeks to see control pain/swelling of ***osteoarthritis***

- ➤ **"*Maxxima*"** – 11 essential oil ext/natural herbs. 25 Euro clinical studies. ↓ pain/triggers body's healing mechanism/↓ inflammation/relax muscles. Biowell

- ➤ **"*JointCare*"** for **rheumatoid** – attack sympt **+** agents w/o side effects. Study shows 78% no pain **+** 52% drop in ESR rating. Himalaya USA 800-869-4640.

- ➤ **Larrea tridentate/Chaparral** – contains lignan NDGA – antioxidant/anti-inflammatory/anti-viral/bacterial. 90% pain relief for *rheumatoid arthritis* w/capsules for 2 wks. *Shegoi* LarreaRX, Inc. www.shegoi.com. (HSI)

- ➤ **Mycoplamas infection** – blood microscopy or PCR-DNA test to identify 800-950-4686. If test positive – Dr. Darryl See treats w/Colloidal silver (see infections) 3-5ppm (max) + Selenium 200-400 mcg + magnesium-peroxide sup.

- ➤ **"*Lyprinol*"** An extract from green-lipped mussels – Eicosate-traenoic Acids (Omega-3 FA) out performs Indomerhacian® for pain/inflame. but doesn't rebuild (Vitamin Shoppe).

- ➤ **Boron** – 3 mg 2x/day relieves many symptoms & inexpensive (Dr Jonathan Wright)

- ➤ **SAMe** – provides raw materials for chemical reactions. 400-600 mg 2 x/day + 800 mcg B_{12}/1,000 mcg folic acid w/meals effective + detox & cartilage formation in some cases but pricey + mood/anxiety improve. (Wright/Stengler)

- ➤ **Wild dog rose rosehips** – Denmark: 66% osteo-arthritis de-creases pain/stiffness after 3 months. *"Litozin"* www.swansonvitamins.com (Prev Mag)

- ➤ **Fish/cod liver/flax oil** – Omega-3 FA = decreases inflame-mation, pain, reverses deteriorated joint cartilage, + lubricate, + decreases BP/cholesterol. 1.8 mg DHA + 1.2 mg EPA or 1 T oil + 400 IU Vit E (mixed tocopherols) 2-3 x/day for <12 wks for results - not w/Coumadin. (Whitaker/Stengler)

- ➤ **Vit C, D, Folate, Magnesium** deficiencies – Dr Osborne

- ➤ **Milk thistle/silymarin** – 2009 Hussain study 320 mg stops the pain cascade

➢ **Evening Primrose Oil** = Omega-6 EFA/GLA – arthritis pain, GLA = inflammation, prev clots, prevent nerve damage from diabetes. Take w/omega-3 oil sup. w/meals. (Stengler)

➢ **"Kaprex"** – oleanolic acid from olive leaf ext./rosemary leaf ext./hops ext/Luduxin. Research data shows may inhibit/reduce PGE2 producing enzymes, stim's circulation to reduce pain/inflammation/protect stomach lining in 7-10 days. (HSI)

➢ **Vit E/Sel/iodine** – osteo/**Kashin-Beck disease**

➢ **Ginger** – for **rheumatoid** & **osteoarthritis** w/2 clinical studies- 75% of patients got relief, inhibits prostaglandins prod.= eases pain/infl. as well as any NSAID/ OTC drugs + improves dig/circulation.. 1-2 g split 2-3x/day w/meals. No Coumadin. (Whitaker/Stengler/ Wilson) **Zinaxin = Ginger extract** – eat root, tea, supplements, extract (Prescription Alt). **Zingiber officialis** – ginger root extract ↓ pain/swelling.

➢ **Cayenne** (capsicum annuum/capsaicin) – standardized cream @ .025-.075% capsaicin 2-4x/day depletes nerves of neuro-transmitter that emits pain messages. (Stengler) 4 week study in Jl of Rheumatology = apply cream 4x/day. Not w/Coumadin. (Dr Wilson)

➢ **Turmeric/Curcumin**. Double-blind studies = reduces pain/stiffness from **rheumatoid/osteo**. + eases symptoms of IBS. 250-500 mg (std 80-90% curcumin) 3x/day. (Wilson)

➢ **Ashwaganda or "Indian Ginseng"** – excellent adaptogen. 1000s of yrs old Ayurvedic remedy for fatigue, memory, asthma, bronchitis, psoriasis, arthritis, stress, anxiety, exhaustion, inflammation, anti-epileptic effect. 1,000-3,000 mg/day (Dr Stengler)

➢ **Cloves** – Chinese medicine lists it as having warming properties for stiff joints/relieving pain when due to cold weather.

➢ **Reconstructive therapy** – treat of a mix of nutrients that stimulates fibroblasts to brings more blood/oxygen/nutrients & stimulates repair of ligaments/tendons/cartilage for **arthritis/carpal tunnel/tendonitis**/etc. (Dr Null)

➢ **Rheumatoid** = desensitize/elim of food allergies – *Dr James C Breneman's book* **Basics of Food Allergy**

➢ **Rhus Toxicodendron** or **Rhus tox** – homeopathic dilution 6C potency 2-3 x's/day for eczema & urticaria. Also for **osteo- & rheumatoid arthritis** if hot water feels better + shingles. See homeopathic practitioner. (Dr Stengler)

➢ **Vit D** – see multi-symptomatic. Linked to 2000 genes – *rheumatic* (several sources)

➢ **Foods**/herbs that reduce inflammation = walnuts, spinach, kale, broccoli, turmeric/curcumin, rosemary, ginger

Asthma

- Am. Academy for Enviro. Med. (aaem.com) = best resource. Long-term use of steroids for asthma can cause liver/kidney damage. Linked to chronic inflammation = see 'healing diets'. OTC pain meds may ↑ risk.

➢ **Boswellia/Frankincense** - 300 mg 3 x's/day for 6 wks = 25% - 70% improved (not replace drugs for severe)

➢ **"Oralmat"** – Secale cereale ext. liquid drops ↓ or eliminates need for drugs = asthma/colds/flu/sinus/allergies. 3 drops under tongue/day (HSI)

➢ **"Phytocort"** – performed comparable to corticosteroid/prednisone w/4 herbs = Sophora flavensis/Ganodema lucidum/Glycyrrhiza uralensis-licorice root/Morinda citrifolianoni. Starts working w/in 2 wks, 3-6 mos full effect. (Dr. Ba Hoang/HSI)

➢ **Ashwaganda** or "Indian Ginseng" – excellent adaptogen. 1000s of yrs old Ayurvedic remedy for fatigue/memory/asthma/bronchitis/psoriasis/arthritis/stress/anxiety/inflammation/exhaustion. 1-3,000 mg/day (Dr Stengler)

➢ **CLA** – 4.5 gm/day of this fatty acid naturally fights the fatty molecules that create inflammation desensitizing without harming your arteries like meds. Bonus: it can also help you gain muscle and slim down, helps with diabetes and provides relief for arthritis...(Mercola)

➢ **Good multi-vit/mins** + extra 50 mg Vit B$_6$ & 100 mg Mag 6+ months = ↓ (Dr J Wright)

➢ **Digestive problem**: do test. Low HCL/pepsin gradually ↑ food allergies/impairs Vit B$_{12}$ prod. = Daily **B$_{12}$ injections** often eliminates wheezing entirely; 1000-3000 mcg methyl B$_{12}$/day & taper off w/in 2-3 wks. Inj. of Mg & B$_6$ during attacks eliminates. Orally = 50-100 mg Vit B$_6$ + 200 mg Mag 3 x's/day can ↓ freq. of attacks.

➢ **Vit D –** see multi-symptomatic. Findings have linked 50% increase in the risk of severe asthma attacks due to low levels of Vit D. (Mercola/Rueters)

➢ **D-Hist –** 40 mil. Americans use - treats root cause w/quercetin/stinging nettles/bromelain/NAC. For many, no more drugs/inhalers necessary w/daily dose. Ortho Molecular Products

➢ **Cordyceps sinensis** – solid reputable research behind it w/placebo-controlled studies = increases stamina, energy levels, & endurance, & reduces fatigue, balances adrenal hormones, treats asthma, chronic bronchitis, & sexual dysfunction. It's become the top selling sport supp. (Stengler)

Athletic performance

➢ **Astaxanthin –** Carotenoid that increases strength/stamina/ endurance, decrease post-exertion recovery time & decrease soreness after physical activity. (Mercola)

➢ **Cordyceps sinensis** – solid reputable research behind it w/placebo-controlled studies = increases stamina, energy levels, & endurance, & reduces fatigue, balances adrenal hormones, treats asthma, chronic bronchitis, & sexual dysfunction. It's become the top selling sport supp. (Stengler)

➢ **Creatine** – research proven amino acid that increases muscle phosphocreatine stores to maintain muscle mass/increases recovery/slows onset of fatigue/gives you more energy especially after turn 40. Excess is excreted. (several sources)

➢ **D-Ribose** – primary carbohydrate for ATP production.
➢ **Deficiencies** – potassium, magnesium, & Vit K

- ➤ **"Endothil-CR"** – ext. of specific strain of green tomatoes. Orig. for muscular atrophy. Now legally being used by high-performance athletes/body builders/etc for its muscle/ strength building prop's = "bodybuilding breakthrough of decade" - safe replace for other performance enhancers. Independent study released Dec 2003. Dr. Daniel Mowrey, Ph.D. Novex Biotech www.Endothil.com + GNC/Rite Aid

- ➤ **"Red Deer Antler Velvet"** – ↑ muscle strength/ nerve impulses/athletic performance/wound healing/regulate BP/ treat arthritis/↓ body fat/inflam./antiviral/tumor prop. Lifestar Millennium, Inc 800-858-7477 (HSI).

- ➤ **Soreness/recovery** = ginger/curcumin/arnica/Omega-3/L-Glutamine (+increase muscle mass). Many

Baldness

- ➤ **Procyanidin B-2** – a compound in apples ↑ # & thickness of hair shafts in six months. Topical.

- ➤ **Cedar** combined w/**lavender** rubbed into scalp = hair growth (at least in women)

- ➤ **DHT inhibitor** – 5-alpha reductase is enzyme produced only in certain cells that transforms testosterone into DHT that kicks in balding process. An African androgen blocker come from African ever-green. "Restore FX" combines 4 blockers + Biotin/ zinc/copper/sulfur-base DL-Methionine, MSM, & L-cysteine, DIM, & Grape seed extract. (NorthStar)

Bladder Infections

- ➤ Women - **estriol cream** + buffered Vit C = 95% success – if due to estrogen drop (New Eng. Jl of Med.)

- ➤ **SSKI** – super saturated potassium iodide; **"Tri-quench"** drink 10-15 drops w/water/juice every 3-4 hrs (no ext. use)

- ➤ **MSM** - fights urinary tract infections + arthritis

- ➤ **Burdock** – for chronic UTIs. Detoxifier = supports liver, destroys blood impurities (bacteria/yeast), helps lymphatic system/digestion/elimination, rich in minerals, phytonutrients + boosts metabolism/healing. 300-500 mg 2-3/day (Stengler)

- ➤ **Cantharis** – homeopathic for burns & urinary/bladder infections. 200C potency (2 x 30C potency 3-4x/day). For UTI, can combo w/antibiotics. (Dr Stengler)

- ➤ **Cranberry juice** w/o sugar (men); **sodium bi-carbonate/** baking soda (women) ¼ t in water & drink

- ➤ **Parsley** – make fresh tea: 1 c/1 qt hot water, cover & steep for 15 mins. Strain & drink 1 cup cooled.

Burns/Sunburns

- ➤ **Cantharis** – homeopathic for burns including severe sunburns, urinary/bladder infections. 200C potency (2 x 30C potency 3-4x/day). For sunburns, dissolve in purified water & spray soln over area. (Dr Stengler)

- ➤ **Tea tree oil** (Melaleuca alternifora oil) = anti-inflammatory/ analgesic/antiseptic/anti-bacterial/fungal/viral for acne/boils/ athlete's foot/**burns**/cold sores/cuts/insect bites/lice/rashes/ warts/gingivitis (gargle). 5% extract cream or gel; as a soap; or 10 drops in 1 t water (not undiluted). Not for infants. (Stengler)

- ➤ **Zinc** – for **burns**/colds/immunity. 45 mg/day. (Dr Stengler)

- ➤ **Aloe vera** – pure; used for centuries topically. Many

- ➤ **L-Glutamine** – IV w/surgery for severe burns + supp afterwards. Dr Osborne

Cancer — (see 'healing diets' in intro)

What is cancer? It is a general term for many chronic diseases characterized by damaged cells that have lost control of reproduction that manifest as different symptoms. Cancer is a multi-faceted complete process that needs an individual treatment plan.

Chronic diseases, including most cancers, are also called diseases of affluence or Western diseases. < 15% of cancers are linked to infections like EBV or hepatitis. But < 97% of all cancers are environmentally induced. **Chronic** inflammation is underlying root cause. *It's not genetics, it is epigenetic* (how genes are expressed/ turned on/triggered)' – Dr Jones. That means < 97% up to you & within your control. Your genes do not determine your fate, your **4 pillars of health - diet, lifestyle, stress, & environment do.**

Mayo Clinic press release, 'no more slash (surgery)/burn (radiation)/ poison (chemo) as it does not work'. Dr Collins "90% of malignancies = environmental factors."

What causes cancer to manifest? **FACTS**: (Dr Darryl Wolfe)

➢ **Cancer is Fungus:** In 1931, Otto Warburg was awarded the Nobel Prize in Science for this discovery. He identified fungus as the causative agent. Cancer cells have mitochondrial ***dysfunction*** & function on **cellular fermentation of glucose** sugars (fungus gives you cravings to feed THEM).

➢ **Cancer epidemic timing**: the introduction of antibiotics in 1950 to kill bacterial infections kills all bacteria.

➢ **Mitochondria:** ancient **bacteria** that reside inside our cells in the 100s or 1000's per cell that make energy for us. **Glyphosate** in 'Round up', a **'probable' carcinogen** that causes free-radical damage that triggers cell mutations was originally patent pending as an antibiotic (kills bacteria) now sprayed on our food to kill plants. Over the last 20 years or so, farmers spray it on all grain crops to kill them before harvest then soak them in it.

➢ **Industrial pollutants** – cars (inside too), smog, beauty shops (dyes, nails,…), print shops, dry cleaning, carpet, petroleum, coal, pesticides, air fresheners, candles, cleaning products, body products (sunscreen, lotions,..), laundry soaps, mold, radon, …

➢ **Compromised immunity** – Everybody produces cancer but not everybody gets cancer. Normally, our immune system recognizes & destroys it. Our gut houses most of our immune system & controls fungal overgrowth. When this immune system is destroyed by antibiotics, etc. & so busy defending us from our environment, this process gets 'de-prioritized' creating the 'perfect storm' for fungus & mitochondrial damage.

➢ **Cancer is a frequency.** Carbs/sugar are not only acidic but addictive, low frequency foods. The affected cells, tissues, organs are your weak link that attracts fungus. **Cancer** is dependent on what you think, eat, drink, & do daily.

Testing:
1. **RGCC Onconomics** plus test (formerly oncostat)/**Greece test**– tests chemosensitivity & herbals for killing your cancer
2. **Mammaprint** – genetic test for early stage breast calculates risks of recurrence/recovery/benefit from chemo or not.
3. **Coloprint** – for colon cancer calculates risk for relapse.

Scans – not mandatory!
- ➢ **CT** – can spot but not detect if is cancer but is 100-1000x's stronger than x-ray's - causes DNA damage/increase risk. + unreliable measuring size + % changes are misleading.
- ➢ **PET** – radioactive glucose uptake; cancer is faster, but so do infections + 1000 x's more radiation than chest x-ray
- ➢ **MRI** – no ionizing radiation so safer
- ➢ **Ultrasound** – can measure
- ➢ **Thermography** – temp changes. Better than mammograms

Blood tests – opt for instead of scans but can have false +

- ➢ **CEA** – broad spectrum tumor marker. Normal is <3
- ➢ **CA 125** – ovarian cancer marker. Normal is 1.9-16.3
- ➢ **CA 15-3** – breast cancer marker. Normal is 7.5-53
- ➢ **CA 19-9** – colorectal, gastric, pancreatic. Normal= 36
- ➢ **PSA** – prostate cancer marker. Normal is <4
- ➢ Heavy metal tests, spectrocell test, micronutrient profile test
- ➢ **DIY tests** –
  - ✓ **Navarro** urine test measures hCG elevated with cancer. Normal is <50
  - ✓ **ONCOblot** – detects 25 types of cancer measures ENOX2 protein
  - ✓ American Metabolic Laboratories: **CA profile** test; 7 tests w/blood & urine (more accurate) can get temp. elevated levels with die off with release of CEA into blood (can mean it's working). Get baseline then wait 30-45 days after start program

Botanicals, etc.
- ➢ **HZ** – Dr. Gold's HZ natural therapy that reverses tumor growth by pinpointing specific liver enzyme responsible for setting off "cachexia" & shuts down enzyme. (HSI)

➤ **Mitochondrial support**: NAC, Acetyl-L-carnitine, Alpha Lipoic Acid (ALA), CoQ10 – taken together*, along with a multi-vitamin + Glutathione, vitamin C, K and D, Creatine, PQQ, zinc, selenium. (Dr Ruscio)

➤ **Probiotics** - Dozens of conditions trace back to gut microbes, including cancer. Recent research shows gut microbes control *antitumor immune responses* & that *antibiotics* alter the composition of immune cells, triggering tumor growth. Certain gut bacteria promote inflammation, which is an underlying factor in virtually all cancers, whereas others quell it. Certain cancers have also been found to have infectious underpinnings. Certain gut bacteria also appear to boost response to anticancer drugs. Some chemotherapy agents rely on bacteria to eradicate the tumor, influence gene expression (on/off).

➤ **Antineoplastons** – new therapy by Dr Burzynski (TX), a gene therapy that turns off oncogenes & turns on cancer suppressor genes now FDA approved. 2Xs result for **brain tumors (25%)** + all others = 50-60% of incurables. (Mercola)

➤ **Insulin Potentiation Therapy** (IPT) – makes chemo 10,000 x's more effective = smaller dose/less side effects.

➤ **AMAS blood test** detects antibodies for any form of cancer or **C-reactive protein (CRP or HSCRP) blood test** – High CRP levels = ↑ risk of colorectal cancer, stroke, & diabetes.

➤ **Graviola extract** – (ACGs) 10,000 x's stronger than chemo (Adriamycin®) w/o side affects. Kills *12 diff. kinds* of cancer (liver/lung/breast/skin/kidney/prostate/colon…) w/o harming good cells. Seeks specific enzyme, attaches, & destroys. Drug Co cover-up for 7 yrs trying to synthesize it. In *prostate*, will cause PSA test to go up at 1st. No pregnant. No combo w/CoQ_{10}/Mg/C/B's). Use w/probiotics/digestive enzymes. New species of mtn Graviola (Anonna montana) may prove even better. "Graviola " & "N-Tense " 700 mg 3-4x's/day (Raintree Nut'ls 800-780-9902). No "N-tense" for estrogen + cancers. "Graviola Max" = both species (HSI)

➤ **Iodine deficiency** – 10-20,000 micrograms of detoxified Io. The Truth about cancer – Dr Brownstein

➢ **Fucozanthin**- A marine carotenoid exerting anti-cancer effects by affecting multiple mechanisms found in *spirulina/chlorella*. *Marine Drugs* 11, no. 12 (December 16, 2013): 5130-147.

➢ **Honokiol** – magnolia officianalis ext. attacks toughest cancers. Asian med for centuries. Animal research shows keeps cancer from creating its own blood supply/angiogenesis + prevent tumor growth/prevents PLD enzyme/toxic to B-CLL cells leads to apoptosis/cancer cell death. It can cross blood-brain barrier = Potential dementia/Alzheimer's - ↑ acetylcholine. **"HonoPure"** (HSI)

➢ **Lactoferrin** – (w/or w/o **Procrit®**) iron-building protein in colostrum/neutrophils release lactoferrin = starves cancer cells, stim's WBC production/signals destruction. Can be combined w/other treatments, ↓ chemo side effects + anti-viral/non-toxic. *"Immunoguard"* (Adv Nut. Pro) 500-1500 mg/day

➢ **IV or liposomal Vit C** – research/studies even w/chemo, lowers side effects/anti-ox. (or caps < 60 gms/day to tolerance)

➢ **Quercetin** (add Vit C) - suppresses cancer cell proliferation, promotes cancer cell apoptosis (programmed death) and mitigates DNA damage. In addition, it has been shown to prevent/slow tumor development in brain, liver, colon. (NH365)

➢ **Lysine/Proline/Proteolytic enzymes** – Amino acids dissolve + enzymes support cell when taken *away from food* to help clean up internally & dissolve cancer proteins. (many)

➢ **Fucoidan/Kombu/Laminaria japonica** – a brown seaweed from Okinawa, Japan. Studies showing it causes stomach/colon/leukemia to self-destruct by physically interfering w/cells ability to stick to tissue (no metastasis) enhances production of macrophages gamma interferon, & interleukins. (HSI)

➢ **Coriolus versicolor** –"hot-water" mushroom ext.; mainstream treatment in Japan/China w/or w/o other treatments for *breast, stomach, colon, lung* (several sources)

➢ *"Peakimmune4"* w/RBAC – *immunity* = triples activity of natural killer cells + increases T & B cells (BRM4). Check w/Dr. for drug interactions & do not take w/immunosuppressant drugs. HF stores.

➢ **SKIN CANCER - BEC5 (Curaderm)** – eggplant ext. (Solanaceae family) cures non-melanoma *skin* cancers in 3 mos. 80,000 cases/26 yrs in use + use for basal/squamous/actinic keratosis. Known since 1825, Royal London Hosp double-blind study = complete regression in 3-13 wks. (Dr White).

➢ **Selenium** increases survival by 51%, cut risks of lung/colon/ prostate by 64% (Bottomline Health).

➢ **Procaine** – *"GH-3/H-3 Plus"* repairs damaged cell membranes to improve nutrient uptake 70%, decreases % get diseases/infections – help w/emphysema/cholesterol/heart disease/*Hodgkin's*/Parkinson's. Covered on 60 min – 100 mil people use. *"Ultra H-3"* 1-2 x/day. Uni Key Health Sys. 800-762-9395 www.unikeyhealth.com.

➢ **AGS** – a glycoside group from sugar given to terminal patients w/86% remission rate – *colon/lung/ovarian/kidney/ brain/pancreatic* cancer. (HSI)

➢ **Lapacho** – studies show Brazilian herb works on cancer = *leukemia/skin/cervical/breast* + anti-viral/bact'l/ fungal. Can drink as tea to prevent colds/flu. (Whitaker)

➢ **Wheat germ extract** – a drink that blocks abnormal glucose uptake in cancer cells starving them to death. 100+ studies proven effective over traditional treatment alone for **lymphoma/pancreatic/breast/lung/prostate/ovarian/ melanoma/colorectal**. (Williams/HSI)

➢ **Astragalus** – 500 mg/15 drops: herb curbs chronic colds, ear infections, & flu, has anti-viral/bact'l/fungal prop's + **prevent/ treat cancer/protects against chemo damage**/ balance sugar & stimulates healing of kidney/nerve damage from high sugar levels/diabetes. Boosts immune fcn by ↑ interferon & T-cells, macrophages, & NK, restores immune fcn in 90% of cancer patients & ↑ twice survival rate. (Stengler/Fuchs)

➢ **Modified Citrus pectin (MCP)**– interferes w/metastasis. Anti-adhesive agent to *cancer cells* (90% reduction) including lymph nodes w/no toxicity. 15 gms/day. (Adv. Nut. Pro 800-232-3536)

➢ **FDA** – approving anti-fungal drugs for cancer – see candida

➢ **Agaricus Blazei Murill (ABM)** – Research w/Brazil mushroom triggers T-cells/interleukin/TNF/macrophages

➢ **Guacatonga** – NCI, Bristol, RTI = all researching clerodane diterpenoids for **mouth/lung/colon/ovarian** cancers. Used for centuries for inflammation/pain/bites w/o side effects. Trials underway for *sarcoma* patients. Free samples may be available if participate in monitoring. Raintree Nut'ls.

➢ **Indole-3-carbinol** (I-3-C) - **broccoli extract** in mustard/ brassica veggies - reverses many cancers/improves 2/16 hydroxyestrogen ratio. 1 study = remission in 12 wks – **cervical/breast/uterine/prostate/lung/colon** (Alternatives). At home test. Any ratio <1.0 is poor. **SSKI** can help – 6-8 drops for 2-3 mo. promotes metabolism of estrone/estradiol into estriol. (Dr J Wright/M Bell, MD study)

➢ **Tetracycline** – antibiotic - blocks enzymes MMP (destroys collagen) & gelatinase-A that helps **prostate/breast** cancer metastasize. (Rowen MD) - take anti-fungal w/this.

➢ **AHCC extract** – Japanese medicinal mushrooms increase immune system, destroys tumor cells, & prevents recurrence: **liver/leukemia/prostate/ovarian/breast cancers/multiple myeloma** w/o side effects. Stimulates cytokine prod/↑ NK cell activity 300%/increases lymphocyte #'s & activity/increases interferon levels (↓ viral/bact'l)/↑ formation of TNF proteins. 3 gm/day = remission in trials. *ImmPower* (Harmony Co.)

➢ **Essiac** – Herbal mixture. Yrs of research reversal of many types of terminal patients to full remission. Best = see an herbalist or Flor-essence drink (low dose)

➢ **Jiaogulan/"Jagulana"** – inhibits tumor growth, normalizes both hi & low BP disorders, strengthens immune system, improves sleep patterns, regulates cholesterol. (HSI)

➢ **L-Glutamine – fuels immune cells, heals Leaky Gut** - A common side effect of chem/radiation, mucositis (inflame. of digestive tract/ulceration to mucous lining. Dr Osborne

➢ **Vitex Agnus Castus** - Test-tube studies; helped kill cancerous colon/stomach/uterus/ovary/breast/cervix/lung. Healthline.com

➢ **DMBQ** – fermented wheat germ effective in reduces chances of recurrence w/chemo. *"Avemar"* 9 gms = 67% ↓ metastasis, 62% ↓ in deaths. + ↓ frequency/fatigue/nausea/ weight loss/immune suppression as cuts off *cancer cell's* energy supply as slows glucose metabolism/keeps from repairing/replicating DNA by reducing PARP enzyme & increase Caspase-3 enzyme to program cell death + *immune-enhancing* properties to fight 2ndary infections by 42%. (wheat allergy) Not w/transplants/fructose intolerance. *Ave"* The Harmony Co. www.theharmonyco.com or Am. BioSciences

➢ *"COBAT/* Taurox SB 6X"** boosts energy (**no Procrit®**) – dev by cancer researchers as combo of 2 AA normalizes/stims immune system increasing some cytokines & decreases others = normalizes. Not w/immuno-suppressors/AI dis. NutriCology

➢ **Wormwood plant ext** – Dr H Lai, U of W – kills skin cancer cells while leaving healthy skin intact. (Williams)

➢ **Hyssop** – effective as an antiviral showing promise for *AIDS/Karposi's sarcoma*

➢ **Vit C/K₃** therapy – addition or alone for *breast/cervix/lung/ colon/liver/stomach*. Generates hydrogen peroxide = kills cancer cells + ↑ sensitivity/effectiveness of other therapies by 14-50% in 2 case studies. Correct ratio 100:1 w/6 gm Vit C/60 mg K₃ daily. K₃ hard to find - *"ProsStay"* (www.life-enhancement.com. Best result *Breast w/* IVA Vit C (Whitaker)

➢ **Melatonin Supp therapy** – not just sleep but strong anti-oxidant for *breast/prostate* cancer - controls excess estrogen (possible culprit). Proven to improve chemo/radiation results as boosts survival odds for metastatic cancer. (several sources)

➢ **Pomegranate juice** – study of 50 men treated for **prostate** cancer = slowed/PSA down. 1 shot/day. (Dr Pantuck/Stengler)

➢ **Colloidal silver** – natural anti-microbial. Swish/gargle/ swallow small amount daily

➢ **"Gerson" therapy** – treatment protocol using huge amounts of fruit/veg juices to supercharge immune system. Mex Clinic.

➢ **Mustard** – U Texas Anderson Cancer Ctr + Univ of Leicester/ Eng (mostly animal studies) = **curcumin** (Indian curry) halts spread of *breast* cancer, makes *chemo* less toxic/**selenium** cuts *prostate* cancer in ½/**isothiocyanates** inhibits growth of existing cancer cells & protective against new. (Dr Inglis)

➢ **Green Tea/extract** – protects/against **breast/liver/lung prostate/esophageal/stomach/colon/bladder/ovarian/ skin cancers**. Antioxidant polyphenols protects DNA from damage & prevents cytochrome P450 enzyme in liver from activating carcinogens during detox. Drink before meals. Add copper, manganese, NAC to shrink capillaries. (TTAC-Rath)

➢ **Concentrated Flax Hull Lignans** - breaks down in colon to enterolactone & enterodial + ALA. **Breast/prostate** - decreases C-erbB2/HER2 protein apop-tosis/free androgen drop/improved BPH symptoms. Promising for **GIST/basal cell skin/bladder/lymphoma/leukemia.** (HSI)

➢ **Turmeric/curcumin** – almost all types/has most evidence-based research for cancer - cell mutation/tumor growth/ metastasis/anti-inflam/prevents angiogenesis, apoptosis. Works synergistically w/some chemo drugs, enhancing it while protective to healthy cells. Helps to alleviate toxic side effects of cancer drugs, while increasing their effectiveness. Integrative MD may recommend curcumin as a comple-mentary chemo treatment. Put it in/on everything – juice, slices, powder/caps w/black pepper ↑ bioavailability 2,000X.

➢ **Quercetin** - Helping prevent cancer cell growth from breast, colon, prostate, endometrial and lung cancers. Modulates immune system, heals leaky gut,… Mercola

➢ **Ginger** – 10,000 times more effective than chemo on cancer stem cells for *breast* cancer. Food Revolution Network.

➢ **The incurables program** – complete hardcore 30 day herbal detox by Dr Schultz done after Clark's cleanse.

➢ **Burdock** - Research shows arctigenin in burdock exhibits cytotoxicity by inducing necrosis in cancer cells + arctiin, demonstrates strong cytotoxic effect on lung/ovarian/skin/ CNS/colon cancer. (Tennent)

➤ **Aloe Vera juice/gel** – 75 active compounds, accelerates gut healing, immune stimulator, anti-microbial (fungus), 6-8 oz/day but can do up to 24 oz/day therapeutic dose

➤ **Beta-glucan or** mushroom extract. Immuno-modulator activates immune response. 1 500 mg/50 lbs body weight. I like fermented turkey tail or rishi.

➤ **Black cumin seed oil** – 100 different compounds/thymo-quinone. Increases natural killer immune cells. Studies show stops proliferation, metastasis, angiogenesis, causes apoptosis (cell death) in dozens of different cancer types. Helps with chemo. 2 T 2x/day & ground/sprinkle/liquid/caps

➤ **FOODS:** Green Med info has assembled list w/>60 articles/studies what foods help kill cancer including drug resistant. **Curcumin/Turmeric** came is 1st (26 studies), **paprika** 2nd (6 studies). **Chlorella** & **Spirulina** daily detox. (Mercola). **Bitter melon** for apoptosis/stops metastasis. (NIH) **Turnips** – great for all cancers particularly colon (Mercola). **Horseradish** (Axe)

Essential oils: 'Only tested on cancer cells in vitro or human testimonials' – DrEricZ,com
- ✓ **Myrrh oil** – anti-cancer prop's increase w/Frankincense
- ✓ **Thyme -** prostate, lung carcinoma, and breast cancers
- ✓ **Citrus oils** – d-limonene has anti-cancer/inhibiting growth
- ✓ **Clary sage oil** – causes apoptosis/cell death in cancer cells
- ✓ **Lavender** – anti-oxidant, support for brain (aroma/bath/diluted onto skin) + calms anxiety
- ✓ **Peppermint/spearmint** – anti-microbial, improves dig.
- ✓ **Oregano** – antioxidant/antimicrobial/anticancer.

➤ **Prevention** – reduces risk of cancer.
- ✓ See 'healing diets'
- ✓ Avoid sugar/glucose – cancer cells need huge amounts.
- ✓ High intake **Vit K2** – EPIC study analyzing over 24,000 participants = 14% less likely to get. Mayo Clinic - same.
- ✓ **Vit A + Folic acid + B$_{12}$ + Zinc + selenium.** **Selenium** deficiency – Indiana Univ. study seeing gene p53 to repair damaged DNA – prevents/repairs

Candida/Yeast infection – secretes 79+ potentially toxic byproducts that tax immune system/drain energy. **Candida/ Keto diet** protocol (see 'healing diets'). Possible link to cancer.

➤ **Candida** – stats <70% US pop infected. Test for antibodies - Candida IgG/IgM. Candida causes extreme fatigue/brain fog/ sugar cravings/mood swings/weight gain/leaky gut triggered food allergies/intolerances/sensitivities/auto-immune cond'ns.

➤ "***Nystatin (prescript)/Candidex/Yeast avenger***" (cleanses) + flaxseed oil/**allicin**-garlic +probiotics + paleo/keto/low carb w/no wheat/yeast/cured meats/cheese/sugar/mush-rooms.

➤ **Rotational botanicals**: Biocidin/Oregano oil/golden-seal/ grapefruit seed ext/pau d'arco = all anti-microbials +probiotics

➤ **Activated coconut/bamboo charcoal/bentonite clay –** Candida loves heavy metals/toxins. Use binds & carries out + toxins & die off reactions. Milk thistle to support liver. (many).

➤ **MCT oil/Undecylenic acid:** (high in caprylic acid) anti-microbial/fungus w/no built up tolerance.

➤ **Enzymes:** Hemicellulase, protease, Cellulase have been shown to break down candida's cells walls/biofilm. Must be in a protective capsule that will not break apart w/stomach acid.

➤ **Siberian fur/tea tree/clove EO/Black Walnut/cat's claw** – + 4 **ringworm/athlete's foot/jock itch/candida.**

➤ **Neem leaf** – Ayurvetic anti-fungal, specific to bad bacterial species/virus' linked esp. to diabetes/eczema/heart disease.

➤ **Vagina infections – SSKI** (super saturated potassium iodide) 20-30 drops in douche 1x/day (5-10 days). If these don't work, try **boric acid capsules** inserted vaginally morning/eve. (Prev)

Carpal Tunnel Syndrome
Has been linked to heavy metals. See 'healing diets' & inflammation

❖ **P5P** form of **Vit B$_6$** 100 mg 3x/day/for 2-3/wks. **DMSO** (liquid rub from HF store; reduces inflam & scar tissue) + liquid **Vit B$_{12}$** (prescription for injectable) mixed & rubbed on w/cotton ball towards heart – 2-3x/day.

Cholesterol

– Studies show lower cholesterol **does not** ↓ heart disease risks, etc. & Statin drugs can cause diabetes (JAMA). Real culprit = inflammation caused by **homocysteine** *(sugar/toxins/ GMOs/leaky gut/pesticides insulin resistance/stress)*. Drugs are obsolete. 200-250 = fine. **Statin drug** manufacturers list side effects – dizziness/liver toxicity/hair loss/constipation/heartburn/mental decline/depletes nutrients - need 100+ mg **CoQ$_{10}$** ....**C-reactive protein test** (CRP) & Lipoprotein (A) tests, Fibrinogen levels, & **omega-3** levels = more deadly heart attack markers. **Hypothyroidism** may be overlooked cause. High w/high triglycerides = too many carbs. High w/normal triglycerides = stress.

➢ **Arjuna** – well-proven cure for lowering LDL/cholesterol + angina attacks w/o side effects (out performed ISMN)+reduces BP & body mass index (wt. loss), atherosclerosis, fight several cancers & bacterial infections. **Cardiac Tonic** (Himalaya USA)

➢ **Policosanol** – safe/natural from citrus peels/sugar cane. Out performs Statins w/o affect to blood sugar. 1 study = Bad chol reduced by 25% & overall chol/LDL reduced 17% + thins blood – intermittent claudication/ ↓ inflam/senility-causing plaques/↑ libido. Interacts w/blood-thinners (HSI/many).

➢ **Red yeast rice extract** – 10 – 13.5 monacolins daily dose; natural form of Lovastatin w/o side effects.

➢ **CoQ$_{10}$** – repairs heart muscle damage, ↓ cholesterol (LDL)/ blood pressure. CoQ$_{10}$ level test. 100-200 mg/day "**CoQMelt**" sublingual = best delivery system = under tongue (many)

➢ **Konjac mannan extract** – lowers BP & cholesterol + blocks fat absorption.

➢ **Pantethine** – vitamin w/new clinical proof to reduces cholesterol/ LDL, increases HDL. (Dr Whitaker)

➢ **Omega 3s (krill or plant based) + Garlic/allicin** – lowers cholesterol, reduce blood pressure, reverse arteriosclerosis.

➢ **Lecithin** – natural plaque-reducer cleans it out & reduces absorption of cholesterol. (Dr David G Williams)

➢ **Niacin** – (no-flush) work up to 2,000 mg will bring up HDL & lower LDL & triglycerides (25+%)

➢ **Chelation therapy** w/**EDTA** - amino acid similar to vinegar – clears out heavy metals + Ca in plaque/joints/ kidneys/ chol-esterol/arthritis/hearing loss. Health Resource "***Enhanced Oral Chelation***" capsules = Vit's/Min's/Aminos. 800-471-4007 Most common dose = 1,000 – 2,000 mg or "***Cardio Clear***" (Health freedom Nut's 800-980-8780 www.hfn-usa.com)

➢ **Tocotrienols** – A type of Vit E – dissolves arterial plaque + ↓ cholesterol/LDL/thins blood in 12 wks w/ "***Care Diem***" to ↓ or stop taking other drugs/therapies. "***PalmVitee***" CompassionNet – stops progression (92%) & seen to reverse atherosclerosis. (25%) (HSI)

➢ "***Cholectin***" – w/150 mg sytrinol & 400 mg phytosterols - blocks absorption of cholesterol & tricks your body into thinking it's absorbed it all w/long lasting results. FDA approved 800 mg/day. www.biocentrichealth.com.

➢ **Cholesterolblock** – Clinical studies at U of Ca - a natural sub. w/o side effects - body mistakes this harm-less soy ingredient for bad cholesterol, absorbs it instead.

➢ **Nitric oxide** – proven effective by Mayo clinic to reduce cholesterol/arterial plaque/expands blood vessels (decrease BP)/controls platelet function/relieves impotency. Contains L-arginine + L-citrulline. (Bottomline Health)

➢ **EPL** – Supplement w/7 int'l studies document plaque melting away, angina gone, EKG's improving, ↓ chol.

➢ **Olive leaf extract** – out performs Captopril in lowering blood pressure + lowers LDL/triglycerides (J Landsman)

➢ **Gugulipid** – this Indian herb boosts low thyroid & lowers cholesterol. (Stengler)

➢ **Berberine** – 27 double-blind, placebo-controlled trials = results to drugs for hypertension/BP drugs, high cholesterol (statins) & Type 2 diabetes (metformin) HSI/Mercola

➢ **Vit K/D3/C**, Mg glycinate, Probiotics, turmeric with black pepper, spirulina, chlorella, modified citrus pectin

> *"Pain & Brain Rescue formula"* – *curcuminoids* from turmeric + Boswellia (inflam.) reduces arthritis, *Gugulipid* burns excess cholesterol/stored fat, increases prostacyclin, cleanses major organs, immune enhancer, anti-bact'l/viral/ fungal, reduces stress/fatigue, *Bioerine* to absorb nutrients in food - better skin/energy. Institute for Vibrant Living

> **Celery** - juice or 4 stalks/day = oil w/*sedanolide* & *butyl phthalide* that relaxes muscles, improves flow, reduces cholesterol/tumors in animals (NE La U School of Pharm)

> **SSKI** – super saturated potassium Iodide; *"Tri-Quench"* dissolves cholesterol. 4-6 drops w/water + niacin/B complex daily + omega's+ methionine + cysteine. Monitor thyroid.

> **Inositol** - diabetic nerve pain, panic disorder, high **cholesterol**, insomnia, cancer, depression, schizophrenia, Alzheimer's disease, ADHD, autism, promoting hair growth, psoriasis.

> **Quercetin** – breaks up calcium deposits, lowers chol/LDL/BP

> **ALA** – breaks up plaque, clears blood vessels, removes oxidized LDL/Cholesterol + lower BP, detox, supports liver (makes chol in defense of inflammation). See more under liver section.

> **Bergamot** – a fruit able to help balance cholesterol levels and LDL, in particular —and other blood lipids. Dr Sinatra

> **B$_6$/B$_{12}$ Vitamins** – helps break down homocysteine that burns artery walls = plaque forms. (several sources)

> **Black cumin seed oil** – studies show reduction (MGB)

> **Fiber** – 30-35 gm total fiber/day reduces triglycerides, homocysteine, & other heart disease markers. (many)

> **Minor** = Grapefruit pectin – 15 gm (Jl. of Clinic Cardiology); Black walnuts – eat 10-12/day; pantetheine, L-carnitine, manganese, betasitosterol, phosphatidyl choline, vanadium, chromium, ginger, **turmeric**/curcumin, fenugreek, rishi mushrooms, garcinia, nuts, spinach, **apples**, cranberries, tomatoes, green tea, fatty fish, beans, capsicum fruit, psyllium, butcher's broom, licorice root, hawthorn berry.

Chronic Fatigue Syndrome (CFS)

(adrenal-function test). High/long stress= adrenals fatigue w/low energy/insomnia/digestion problems/osteoporosis/inflammation leading to dangerous conditions (arthritis/heart disease). Associated w/high cortisol output falling off starting @ age 45. Classic symptoms of adrenal insufficiency = low BP, low blood sugar, chronic inflammation, dehydration/low blood sodium, heavy metals, EMF, underlying/weakened immune system/infection.

➢ **Glutathione** (GSH) -tripeptide of cysteine/glutamine/glycine offers antioxidant protection, reverses fatigue/↑ immune function/detoxifies to combat oxidative/neuromuscular diseases. GHS precursor, cysteine, derived from milk whey is body's preferred form. GHS depletion is core of CFS & strong antiviral. "*CysteinePeP*" NutriCology www.nutricology.com

➢ **DHEA** test (15 mg/day), Cortisol, extra salt (prod of aldos-terone) to regulate potassium/sodium, + good multi. Those w/weak adrenals not best on low-carb. 6+ pieces of licorice (w/o sugar) to slow liver's breakdown of steroid hormones.

➢ **Alpha-lipoic acid** (ALA) – reliable research. Check interactions. Diabetics = 600-1,200 mg/day for 4 wks. Neuropathy = 600-1,200 mg/day for 3-5 wks. For **CFS**/glaucoma/liver disease = 300-1,200 mg/day. (several sources)

➢ **SAMe** (butanedisulfonate form w/enteric coat) – 400-1200 mg/day treats low energy characterized in fibro-myalgia/**chronic fatigue syndrome** & maintain glutathione (antioxidant that supports liver). Any HF Store (HSI)

➢ **Candida/yeast/mold overgrowth** – can be an underlying cause stressing the adrenals with mycotoxins. See candida.

➢ **Sulfur** – homeopathic = cellular detox brings energy back when fatigued, + detox's digestive tract (ulcers/ diarrhea/ flatulence/ IBS), relieves skin ailments. Deficiency sym.= always warm, sweats easily, no blankets, thirsty + likes sweet, spicy foods, fats, & beer. 2 - 6C potency tabs 2/day for 2 weeks. (Dr Stengler)

➢ **D-Ribose** – 150 peer-reviewed published studies on how this carbohydrate is used in ATP energy production. (Weil+)

➢ **Beta-glucan** – mushrooms. Most ailments = micro-infections. Boosts immunity: many chronic ailments –arthritis/ **chronic fatigue**/HIV/herpes/cold/flu/allergies/parasitic/ bacterial infections. "***Immutol***" www.immunocorp.com

➢ **Rhodiola &/or Ashwaganda** or "Indian Ginseng" adaptogens. 1000s of yrs Ayurvedic remedy – fatigue, memory, asthma, bronchitis, psoriasis, arthritis, stress, anxiety, exhaustion, inflammation. Start slow 300 to 3,000 mg/day (Dr Stengler)

➢ **Licorice Root** – Ayurvedic/Chinese med = harmonizing herb. Detox liver/**support adrenals** (burnout)/anti-inflam. (stops prostaglandins)/**chronic fatigue**. High dose side effects - sodium/water retention = increased BP, not w/kidney issues/ hypokalenia, diuretics/digitalis. 1,000 – 3,000 mg/day (Stengler)

➢ **Iron deficiency** – 1 in 4 US women = leading cause between 15-50 due to monthly loss in menstrual blood. Mild deficiency is linked to PMS/depression/impaired fertility/pregnancy complications. Due blood test serum ferritin. (Carlson-Rink, RD)

➢ **EMF/Wifi** – can also be interpreted by the body as a stressor.

Constipation (may be gut dysbiosis issue = probiotics)

➢ **Fiber (60 gm/day)** – on any diet, don't get enough. Sprinkle **flaxseed meal/chia seeds/hemp seeds** on food, smoothies, into sauces. Good source of omega-3s. 1-2 T/meal. (several)

➢ **Cascara Sagrada** – a strong laxative, also treats gallstones, liver ailments, & cancer. Soothe w/aloe vera. (several)

➢ **Slippery elm/Aloe Vera leaf/Caster oil** – alone or together. Remedy for the symptoms of chronic GI problems - leaky gut, ulcerative colitis, Crohn's disease, IBS. Dr Wm Cole

➢ **Vit C or L-glutamine** – high dosages move bowels 2-4 gm/day or to 'bowel tolerance'.

➢ **Magnesium** (oxide or citrate) Supplement therapy – for short-term relief 1,200 mg in divided doses/day. (Dr Stengler)

➢ **Foods** = Avocadoes = 12 g, raspberries/blackberries = 8g, acorn squash = 6 g, black beans = 8 g, sweet potato = 5 g.

Cysts/lipomas (benign tumors made up of solid fat)

➤ **SSKI** (super saturated potassium iodide)**/DMSO** – 50/50 mix rub on w/cotton ball towards heart 2x/day for 2-3 wks. DMSO natural liquid approved by FDA that works as a carrier through the skin. Also decreases inflammation/pain/clears scar tissue. "*Tri-Quench*" Scientific Botanicals or most health food stores. Warning: SSKI continuous use can slow thyroid function.

➤ **Breast/Ovarian Cysts**- fibrocystic/painful breasts & ovarian cysts. Monitor thyroid. **SSKI** – potassium iodide; interacts w/estrogens to metabolize Estrone & 16-alpha-hydroxy-estrone (dangerous form). 6-8 drops/day in water & drink 3-6 mos. (mild – moderate). Severe breasts = **Lugol's** iodine soln applied to vaginal area & cervix followed by magnesium sulfate injection (referral ACAM)

➤ **Cat's claw** – "..rids body of resistant strep frequently misdiagnosed as yeast/Candida. Strep is also true cause of many symptoms/conditions – candida/**cystic acne**/.... + strengthening immune system ..." (medicalmedium.com)

Depression – no Prozac®. Anti-depressants may increase heart disease risk. (Mercola) Also linked to psycho-somatic disorders (Dr Sarno). Check for candida/hormones/dysbiotic microbiome/leaky gut/liver can all contribute/cause.

➤ **S-adenosylmethionine** (AdoMet) – 38 studies proven effective by increases dopamine/serotonin/serotonin/norepinephrine improving the way brain cells receive these chemicals + helps w/liver problems/fatigue/memory/pain & stiffness. (Stengler)

➤ **Tryptophan/tyrosine/phenylalanine** – try before St John's Wort; Amino acids help balance monitored deficiencies. (www.acam.org for referral)

➤ **SAMe** (butanedisulfonate form w/enteric coat) – 38 studies compared to drugs. Treats depression by contributing to production of dopamine/serotonin + helps w/low energy in fibromyalgia/CFS & maintain glutathione (anti-oxidant for liver). 400-1200 mg/day. Not w/Bipolar (HSI/Stengler)

➤ **St John's Wort** – better than Prozac® but try above 1st. (Dr Whitaker) (Dr Stengler recommends this 1st).

- **Procaine** – "*GH-3/Ultra H-3*" repairs damaged cell membrane = improve nutrient uptake 70%, ↓ % get diseases – help w/depression/heart dis. Covered on 60 min – 100 mil people. "*Ultra H-3*" 1-2 x/day Uni Key Health Sys. (HSI)

- **Bipolar** – natural protocol = **Fish oil** w/EPA & DHA 2,000 mg/day + **B₁₂** 1,000 mcg + **Folic acid** 800 mcg/day (Stengler)

- **Ignatia** – for depression brought on by grief/disappointment/stress/tension headaches. Many psychologists & counselors have observed quicker recovery/big changes in outlook. 30C 2/day for a week (Stengler)

- **Inositol** - used for diabetic nerve pain/panic disorder/high cholesterol/insomnia/**depression**/schizophrenia/ Alzheimer's disease/side effects of medical treatment with **lithium**

- **5-HTP** + B Vit's = nat'l amino acid that's converted to serotonin in brain for depression. (Dr Bralch/Stengler)

- **Lion's Mane** – Stim's NGF/regenerates nerves/reduces plaque. GreenMedInfo

- **Withania** – India 3,000+ yrs; treat stress/fatigue/improved memory/blood sugar/cortisol/anxiety/ depression. 47 different beneficial compounds w/studies it's effective. (Stengler)

- **Rhodiola** (roseroot) adaptogen – used for decades. 180+ studies improves short-term memory/concentration/audio-visual perception/alleviates stress-induced insomnia/stress/ **depression**/irritability/hypertension/ headaches. (Lark)

- **"Artic weed"** eat/steep in tea – increases serotonin levels in the brain by 30% to reduce depression, gives energy boost, & helps loose weight. Russian studies since 1970's. (Dr Inglis)

- **Microbiome/dysbiosis issue** – probiotics to re-establish gut flora to make neurotransmitters, GABA, serotonin,….

- **Exercise** - "Molecular biologists/neurologists have begun to show that exercise may alter brain chemistry in much the same way that antidepressant drugs do -- regulating the key neurotransmitters serotonin & norepinephrine."

Detox –

Our toxic load from heavy metals/pesticides/herbicides/etc. is higher than ever in human history - More than what the body can handling. The body will do as much as it can w/liver, gut bacteria, skin, kidneys, & colon, throwing the excess into fat storage, some leaks out of the intestines into the blood, crosses the blood brain barrier & a variety of symptoms manifest.

Many different types of detoxing/cleansing protocols – liver/gall-bladder w/olive oil, colon w/cascara, aloe, & leaky gut protocol,…..

The bacteria in fermented foods that detox pesticides: Leuconostoc mesenteroides WCP907, Lactobacillus brevis WCP902, Lactobacillus plantarum WCP931, Lactobacillus sakei WCP904, (& other ferments + fulvic/humic acid) utilize them as sole source of carbon/phosphorus. (Jl Ag Food med)

Detox support: There are phases (Also see heavy metals & liver)
➢ **Liver:** milk thistle, dandelion root, NAC, ALA, selenium, glutathione, B's, copper, zinc, Vit c/E/D/CoQ10, ….
➢ **Binders:** taken away from food/supplements - modified citrus pectin (MCP), zeolite/bentonite clay, coconut or bamboo charcoal (comes in different sizes for different goals)
➢ **Chlorophyll:** phytoplankton, cilantro, spirulina, chlorella.
➢ **Foods:** garlic, onions, ginger, broccoli sprouts, egg yolks, beets
➢ **Others:** 'Biosil', **Calcium D-Glucarate** (CDG), silica,…

Diabetes – It is NOT your fault! The failed food pyramid of
high grains & low fat & our toxic food supply is. High blood sugar damages all organs/tissues for everyone + liver congestion/NAFLD (see liver, weight loss, & healing diets sections).

✓ Get off plastic bottles – BPA leakage = rapid spikes insulin
✓ No more Glucophage®/Acarbose®/Metformin or Statin drugs now linked to cause other conditions (JAMA).
✓ Discuss alternatives/monitor w/Dr. these drugs for several wks/months then ↓ drugs over time to eliminate w/diet.
✓ **Chronic inflammation/Autoimmune/leaky gut/ thyroid =** underlying root causes to allergies/insulin resistance/ metabolic syndrome/arthritis/diabetes/ osteoporosis/heart disease/cancer.

➢ **Konjac mannan extract** (replace Acarbose®) controls sugar + blocks fat absorption, lowers BP & cholesterol

➢ **Agarcius Blazei** – medicinal mushroom that boosts adiponectin levels to normalize insulin efficiency + relieves stress/boost immunity/healthy cholesterol. (HSI)

➢ **MHCP** = Cinnamon ext stabilize blood sugar. Study = 500 mg 3x/day. *Cinnulin PF* or *"Insulife"* – MHCP + chromium. (Dr Jonathan Wright/HSI +) *"Glucotor 2"* – 82% effective, boosts body's insulin response, w/ *Cinnulin PF* - 300% more effective w/o toxic side effects + improved cholesterol (Baseline Nut)

➢ **Modified citrus pectin** – detox Arsenic – from water, rice, …interfering w/pancreas insulin production. Myers

➢ **Cinnamon cassia** - helps w/metabolic syndrome (abdominal fat/high blood sugar/BP). USDA study 1-6 g/day (1/4 -1 tsp) for 40 days lowered glucose & triglycerides by about 25% + reduced LDL up to 27%. (Dr Winston/Fuchs)

➢ **Vit D** – linked to 20,000 genes = low levels linked to immunity/ type 2 diabetes/asthma/ depression/cancer. 28 studies/100,000 people = High levels ↓ risk. Recommendations now run about 5K – 10K/day. (Mercola + other sources)

➢ *"MetaPhase"* – curbs cravings/↓ blood sugar/ reverses metabolic syndrome/repairs damage. Yrs of clinical studies (China) – circulatory/cholesterol/athero-sclerosis/heart disease/nerve damage/ restoring organ/endocrine function. HSI - www.puretango.com

➢ **Serratiopeptidase** (SP) *"Arthro Enzyme"* from silk moths = blocks pain by stopping release of pain-causing Amines from inflamed tissues/drains harmful fluids/shrinking swelling/ speeds tissue repair/cleans up metabolic wastes/dissolves dead/ damaged tissue, **diabetic neuropathy**. Used in Europe for 23+ yrs - Jl of Internal Med 40 clinical studies.

➢ **Selenium Deficiency** - also affects thyroid (Hyman)

➢ **L-Glutamine** – heals leaky gut/leaky brain, stops sugar cravings,…. Dr Osborne

➢ **TYPE 1**: Vit D deficiency,….Dr Osborne

➢ **5-HTP** – an amino acid that curbs sugar cravings by increasing serotonin brain levels. 50-100 mg 2x/day on empty stomach. No anti-depressants (Dr Stengler)

➢ **Berberine** – outperforms Metformin in studies. Shown to reduces blood sugar/cholesterol/LDL/BP/triglycerides/ boosts AMP-K. DrMurry.com +

➢ **Gymnema Sylvestre** – staves off sugar cravings/balances blood sugar. In test subjects, ↑ in # of pancreatic insulin secreting beta cells – repair/regenerate new cells, ↑ activity of enzymes responsible for glucose uptake/utilization. Researchers found in 1 control study w/**Type I diabetes**, insulin require- ment fell dramatically. **Type 2** study - pancreas ↑ release of insulin & reduced med's. 24-25% gymnemic acids 400-600 mg/day. (Dr Stengler/ Fuchs) *"Advanced Blood Sugar Soln"* = combo cinnamon/chromium/banaba leaf ext/**Gymnema Silvestre**/fenugreek/bitter melon/policosanol. Hlth Res./HSI

➢ **LGB** – codename for type 2 permanent cure in as little as 1 hr w/o drugs by correcting the way body metabolizes food. Univ Pittsburg Dr P Schauer – 83% of obese patients saw improvement/reversal. (+Whitaker)

➢ **Banaba plant** – lowers blood sugar by 32% in 3 wks for mild-mod Type II + lose weight. Active ingredient = coro- solic acid. *Glucosol/Normalose* 48 mg/day. (HSI)

➢ **Mulberry seed extract** – 1 gm/day for 2 months dropped fasting blood sugar 30 pts

➢ **Evening Primrose Oil** = omega-6 EFA/GLA –*diabetic neuropathy*, arthritis pain, inflammation, prevent nerve damage when taken w/omega-3 oil sup. w/meals. (Stengler)

➢ **Dehydroepiandrosterone** (DHEA) - cuts insulin resistance & burns fat; natural to body but production falls off as age. Do test to see if low & supervised by Dr (Dr. Stengler)

➢ **Black cumin seed oil/powder** – studies show lowers blood sugar when consumed (MGB)

> **PGX** – soluble fiber complex that gels/slowing gastric emptying to slow down carb absorption/increases satiety-feel full/increases insulin sensitivity/appetite control

> **Biotin/Chromium** – 2 of most research nutrients for sugar support. Double-blind trial = biotin ↑ 2 specific glucose-metabolizing enzymes – ACC & PC. Chromium research shows could reverse impaired glucose metabolism. (HSI)

> **Vanadium** – confirmed studies that trace mineral could fix fasting blood sugar & remove need for all drugs. Consult w/Dr as may drop too fast. (Dr Whitaker)

> **Quercetin** – a bioflavonoid in apples/onions/berries that reduces enzyme aldose reductase by ½ - studies show causes **diabetic retinopathy** by damaging blood vessels in retina + converts blood sugar to sorbitol. + heals leaky gut, modulates immune system, detoxes radiation. 1,000 mg 3X's/day. (Stengler)

> **Alpha-lipoic acid** (ALA) – reliable research helps improve/stabilize blood sugar/relieve **neuropathy** (type 2) & helps nerves regenerate. Sustained release preferred. Check interactions. 600-1,200 mg/day for 3-5 wks. (several sources)

> **Ginkgo Biloba** – terpene lactones -bioflavonoids/ antioxidants ↑ circulation to the brain, + cataracts, macular degeneration, & **diabetic retinopathy**, ↓ inflammation, relieves varicose veins, & thins blood (↓ BP). 120-360 mg/day. Not w/Coumadin/aspirin. (Dr Stengler)

> **Thiamine/B1** – small amounts prevent/may help reverse damage already done. Recent studies - fat/lipid-soluble form = **Benofotiamine** which boosts cell enzyme **transketolase** that body absorbs about 5X's faster & passes directly though cell membrane. Dr Brownlee applied to FDA. Concerns – rapid plaque removal. (HIS/Wm Campbell – "**GlucoComplete**")

> **Broccoli sprouts** – sulforaphane, a compound found to effectively lower blood sugar levels, assisting those with the disease and helping others to avoid type 2 diabetes.

➤ **Inositol** - is used for **diabetic nerve pain,** panic disorder, high cholesterol, insomnia, cancer, depression, schizophrenia, Alzheimer's disease, ADHD, autism, promoting hair growth, a skin disorder called psoriasis, and treating side effects of medical treatment with **lithium**

➤ **Withania** – used in India 3,000+ years to treat stress/fatigue/ chronic disease/improved memory/blood sugar/cortisol/blood fats/depression. 47 beneficial cmpds found effective. (Stengler)

➤ **Garlic** – glycation threatens eyes, kidneys, skin, blood vessels. Univ of Manchester/England studied special form of 2 yr aged garlic extract that may help stop glycation. (Dr Inglis)

➤ **Pycnogenol** – Univ Italy study = alleviates swelling/edema for diabetes & varicose veins. Can take w/BP meds. (Dr Stengler)

➤ **Hypoglycemia** = "*Glykos*" - a glucose control tablet that reduces sugar cravings, highs, & crashes (www. pachealth.com) or **apple cider vinegar** – 2 T before each meal or pills 2/day.

➤ **Ghee** – butyric acid feels good bacteria, insulin sensitivity, stabilizes sugar.

➤ **Nut butters** – Study 83,000 nurses = 20% lower risk.

➤ **Bitter melon** - better insulin sensitivity/glucose tolerance/ insulin signaling/support weight loss (MSKCC.org)

➤ **Inulin/polyphenols/beta-glucans** – nourish good micro-biome, insulin sensitivity in studies: dandelion & chicory root, asparagus, blueberries, cranberries, red grapes,…Erick Cervantes Fernandez

➤ **Vit K** – helps with neuropathy, mitochondrial function for insulin resistance & rescue dying mitochondria to restore cell. Foods – kale/broccoli/cabbage,…

➤ **Prevent type 2** =
  ✓ Daily doses of Black tea, Sunlight (vit D), turmeric, nuts, chia seeds, green leafy vegetables, apple cider vinegar, cinnamon, red grapes, broccoli, spinach, green beans, and berries.

✓ 90% of all cases of diabetes can be resolved by eating foods rich in nutrients (that's not grains) with a low glycemic load (paleo/ketogenic) and pursuing both weight/burst training and aerobic exercise. (several)

Diabetic good/bad use of sweeteners

Aspartame – *Equal & NutraSweet*
➢ 61 reported adverse rxns/side affects – chest pains/ asthma/ arthritis/migraines/seizures/nerve damage (mimics Parkinson's), etc + stimulates carbohydrate cravings. Breaks down into formaldehyde at body temp.

Sucralose – *Splenda*
➢ Not zero calories, made w/chlorine (toxic). Can't be metabolized/kidney stress/stomach pain/immune system disorders.

Saccharine – *Sweet 'n Low*
➢ Can't be metabolized, linked to cancer, may promotes weight gain (Texas U Health Science Ctr 8 yr study).

Stevia (good)
➢ Brazil/Asia, used for centuries – suppresses glucose response (diabetes II), may reduce blood sugar levels, lower BP, prevent cavities/reduce plaque w/no affects. Some have bitter after taste – 300 x's sweeter than sugar = use 1/6th-1/8th tsp.

Lo Han Kuo/Monk fruit (good)
➢ Momoedica grosvenori. Used for centuries to treat coughs/ sore throats/skin/digestion issues. Natural sweetener 250+ x's sweeter than sugar w/o Cal & heals. Maintains insulin/ blood sugar/↑ bone density/anti-microbial/decreases BMI.

Erythritol (good)
➢ Looks/taste/measure close to sugar but sugar alcohol but w/ ¼ calories, no know side effects.

Xylitol (good)
➢ Looks/tastes like sugar but ½ calories. OK'ed by FDA as additive = good for beverages/baking (not w/yeast), lowers cavity-causing plaque, strengthens tooth enamel, reduces decay by up to 80% (in toothpaste/mouthwash/ gum).

Eczema

Eczema – auto-immune = 'impaired barrier function from 'leaky gut' to 'leaky skin'. Several possible causes – inability to process EFA GLA, food sensitivities/allergy, or Candida/fungal overgrowth. Best food protocol – see 'healing diets' (AIP)

➢ **Fungal** - oregano oil + goldenseal + grapefruit seed ext + pau d'arco + probiotic + fish oil +fiber + Zinc. (Stengler/HSI)

➢ **Burdock** – Detox = supports liver, destroys blood impurities (bact'l/yeast), clears lymphatic system; improves digestion/ elimination. Rich in minerals, phytonutrients, & stimulates healing. 300-500 mg 2-3/day (Stengler)

➢ **Evening Primrose Oil** = omega-6 EFA/GLA = ↓ inflammation, prevents clots. **Eczema** = 26 British clinical trials - 150-400 mg GLA (1,500-3,000 mg oil) + omega-3 oil supplement w/meals. (Dr Stengler) or **DHA** 5.4 gm/day.

➢ **Probiotic** prevents in children.

➢ Natural creams w/**chamomile** as effective as hydrocortisone cream. (Erickson)

➢ **Sulfur** – homeo = cellular/digestive tract detox relieves skin ailments (psoriasis/**eczema**). Deficiency sym.= always warm/ sweats easily/no blankets/thirsty/likes sweet/spicy foods. 2 - 6C potency tabs 2x/day for 2 wks. Skin may flare up temporarily. (Stengler)

➢ **Rhus Toxicodendron** (Rhus tox)– homeo dilution 6C potency 2-3 x's/day. Use in hot water feels better. See homeo practitioner. (Stengler)

➢ **Licorice Root** – Ayurvedic/Chinese herb. Suppress cough/ anti-inflammatory. (stops prostaglandins)/boost viral inter- feron/heal digestive tract (IBS/ulcers), **topical for eczema/ psoriasis**. High dosage can have side effects - sodium/water retention = ↑ BP, no for kidney problems/ hypokalenia, not w/diuretics/digitalis. Tincture drops = 10-30 2-3x/day. Caps = 1,000-3,000 mg/day (Dr Stengler)

➢ **Neem leaf/oil** – ayurvedic for candida

➢ **Tamanu oil/Calophyllum inophyllum** – see psoriasis.

Emphysema – step 1 = test for allergies (see allergies) = produces excess mucus

➢ **Magnesium citrate** – 200 mg 2 x's/day as broncho-dilator + 250 mg **L-carnitine** 3 x's/day for breathing muscles + 500 mg **N-acetylcysteine** 2 x's/day loosens/ thins secretions + **SSKI** 6 drops in drink + 500 IU **Vit A** + 2000 mg **Vit C** + 2 19-grain caps. of **lecithin** + Vit E, copper, & zinc w/Dr's care (Dr J Wright).

➢ **Glutathione inhaler** – 2-3/day (prescription & compound pharmacy)

➢ **Procaine** – "*GH-3/H-3 Plus*" repairs damaged cell membranes to improve nutrient uptake 70%, reduces % get diseases, reduces infections – help w/acne/ arthritis/depression/**emphysema**/ cholesterol/ heart disease/ Hodgkin's/ migraines/MS/osteoporosis/ Parkinson's. Covered on 60 min – 100 mil people use. "*Ultra H-3*" 1-2 x/day Uni Key Health Sys. 800-762-9395 www.unikeyhealth.com.

Epilepsy

➢ **Gotu Kola** – agitation/anxiety/insomnia/epilepsy/ hyperactivity (2 much = rash + sedate)

➢ **Ashwaganda** or "Indian Ginseng" – excellent adaptogen. Ancient 1000s of year old Ayurvedic remedy for fatigue, impotency, memory, asthma, bronchitis, psoriasis, arthritis, stress, anxiety, exhaustion, inflammation, **anti-epileptic effect**. Only a few human studies so far. 1,000-3,000 mg/day (Dr Stengler)

➢ **Ketogenic** dietary protocol – see 'healing diets'

Erectile dysfunction

➤ **L-arginine** – 3-6 gm/day; Amino acid ↑ **nitric oxide** levels. Foods = grains/seed/beans/nuts/chocolate. (No if cancer/herpes) (Whitaker) + 1,200 mg **Cordyceps sinensis** & 30C potency **Lycopodium** 2x/day (Stengler)

➤ **Testosterone deficiency/Nitric oxide** – proven eff by Mayo clinic to ↓ chol/arterial plaque/expands blood vessels (BP ↓)/controls platelet fcn/**relieves impotency**. Contains **L-arginine** + **L-citrulline**. (Bottomline Health). **L-carnitine** – clinical studies in Urology Publication out-performed "little blue pill" & testosterone therapy when usual dosage was ↑ = more energy/better erectile function. (Dr. Whitaker).

➤ **Vit D/Zinc/DHEA** deficiencies (Mercola/Hyman)

➤ **Ashwaganda** or "Indian Ginseng" – excellent adaptogen. Ancient 1000s of year old Ayurvedic remedy for fatigue/**impotency**/asthma/bronchitis/psoriasis/arthritis/stress/anxiety/exhaustion, inflam. Only a few human studies so far. 1,000-3,000 mg/day (Dr Stengler)

➤ **"Argi-Vive III"** = 3,000 mg of L-arginine + Ashwagandha root/Guta cola leaf/horny goat weed/maca root all as a effervescent, berry-flavored drink. (HSI) NorthStar Nut'ls

➤ **Yohimbe** – 18 –100 mg split over 3 x's/day; all natural herb FDA approved (Dr Jonathan Wright)

➤ **Muira puama** 1000-1500 mg/day + **ginseng** 100 mg 2-3/day + **ginkgo biloba** 40 mg 3 x's/day (Dr White)

➤ **Ram's horn/Fenugreek** – contains cmpd saponins glycosides found in studies to increases desire & performance. (HSI)

➤ **Green oat straw** – homeopathic remedy called ultimate aphrodisiac for both men & women. No hormones, drug, stimulant or dilator but raises body's testosterone.

Flatulence - can be associated with IBS/SIBO treated with low FODMAP dietary protocol.

➤ **Sulfur** – homeopathic = cellular detox brings back energy when fatigued, detox's digestive tract (ulcers/diarrhea/IBS/ **flatulence**), & skin ailments. Deficiency sym.= always warm, sweats easily, no blankets, thirsty + likes sweet, spicy foods, fats. Other applications = headaches/hot flashes/insomnia/ sore throat. 2 - 6C potency tabs 2/day for 2 weeks. For skin = may flare up temporarily due to detox. (Stengler)

➤ **Probiotics** – Microbiome dysbiosis corrected

➤ **Chamomile tea** - before bed relaxes bowel/↓ spasms

➤ **Ginger** - 500 mg – antispasmodic; ↓ force/freq. contraction

➤ **Fennel seeds** – calms upset stomach/↓ gas (eat)

Glaucoma/cataracts/macular degen. (MD)

➤ **MD** = considered a digestive problem w/↓ levels of HCL/pepsin. IV inj. until digestion tests are normal. Then, all oral. Zinc & selenium + all ess'l minerals + Vit B_{12} + B-complex halts/reverses about 70%.

✓ **Step 1**=digestion tested/replacement therapy of betaine hydrochloride - pepsin or glutamic-acid hydrochloride-pepsin 1 cap/day (5/7 ½/10 grains) before meals 2-3 days. If no problems, 2 caps/day & continue to gradually ↑ to 40-90/meal. Monitored by Dr. (www.acam. org).

✓ **Step 2**= 30 mg **zinc** 2 x's/day; 4 mg **copper** diff. times than zinc; 1000 mg **taurine** between meals; 800 IU **Vit E;** 300 mcg **selenium**; 80 mg **bil-berry** 2 x's/day. Expect several months before any signs - needs to build up. Since 1985, Dr J Wright =70% success for "incurable" dry MD.

➤ **Hyaluronic Acid** (HA) deficiency – rooster comb ext.; stops breakdown of joint collagen from enzyme Hyaluronidase that attacks HA - lubricates/↓ pain/inflam./protects synovial fluid/repair-restores joint collagen, **macular degeneration**. 9000 reports. "*Alliviate*" = HA + Boswellin, ginger, white willow extract, Vit C Inst for Vibrant Living 800-218-1379

➢ **Goji/Ningxia Wolfberry** – 100+ yrs old; China/Japan/ Tibet. Antioxidant w/zeanthin+carotenoids = ↑ WBC/hemoglobin/ eyes/liver/ kidneys/immunoglobulin A/↓ tumor growth/ **cataracts**/LDL/plaque/BP/fat composition/ blood sugar. "*OCS-147*" combined w/selenium (flush toxins) + turmeric (inflam) + B complex (homocysteine) - BioNutrigenics, Inc

➢ **Cataract eye drops** – dev by Dr Rowen MD states "call compounding pharmacy & request formulation DMSO 6.25% + glutathione 1.25%+Vit C 1.25%". Reverses/prev. 30 sec sting.

➢ **Cataracts = Vit A** – 40,000 IU liquid "micellized"; &/or **N-acetyl-carnosine** (NAC) eye drops; **Hachimi-jio-gan** 150 mg 2 x's/day for early 60% some regression/20% halted; **Bilberry** w/25% std. anthocyanidin 80-160 mg 3 x's/day stopped progression. (Dr J Wright)

➢ **Lutein** (15 mg/day) + **Zeaxanthin** (3 mg/day) + **Zinc** (10-45 mg/day) + **Vit C** 2,000-3,000 mg/day w/meals for **macular degeneration**. To prevent; 2-5 mg lutein/day + 500 mcg Zeaxanthin (several sources)

➢ **Resveratrol** –*Moravian* red wine ext.= *French Paradox*; anti-aging, ↓ blood clots/bad chol/plaque deposits/balance hormones/**macular degeneration**/ COX-2 inhibitor/ rejuvenates/immunity/correct existing condition/ diseases. Harvard/Boston/Yale/N Western… "*Vinotol*"– BioNutrients; "*Botanical Vitality*" Great Life Labs

➢ **Ginkgo Biloba** – terpene lactones -bioflavonoids/anti-oxidants prev/treat Alzheimer's increases circulation to the brain, + strokes, **cataracts/macular degeneration,** diabetic retinopathy, protects blood vessels, reduces inflam, relieves varicose veins, reverse cardiovascular disease, thins blood (↓ BP). 120-360 mg/day. Careful w/Coumadin/aspirin. (Stengler)

➢ **Sulforaphane** – an organic sulfur compound found in cruciferous vegetables – cabbage/broccoli/.. research shows extraordinary potential for protecting fragile retinal cells involved in AMD even promote regeneration, supports detox, & cancer prevention. Nutrition news 2018

- ➢ **Forskohlin** – decreases pressure inside eyes, increases blood flow, + reduces blood pressure (Pres. Alt)

- ➢ **Alpha-lipoic acid** (ALA) – reliable research helps improve/ stabilize blood sugar/relieve neuropathy (type 2). Check interactions. Diabetes = 600-1,200 mg/day for 4 wks. For **Neuropathy** = 600-1,200 mg/day for 3-5 wks. For **glaucoma** = 300-1,200 mg/day. (several)

- ➢ **Quercetin** – a bioflavonoid found in apples/onions/berries that ↓ enzyme aldose reductase by ½ that studies show causes **cataracts**/diabetic retinopathy by damaging retina vessels + converts blood sugar to sorbitol. 1,000 mg 3X's/day. (Stengler)

Gout - a form of arthritis by some; linked to autoimmunity.

- ➢ **Sweet cherries** – Gout attacks are caused by body's inability to get rid of uric acid. Eat 45 fresh Bing cherries for breakfast & after several hrs, blood levels dropped 14% & urine uric acid output increased 70%. (HSI)

- ➢ **Rhododendron caucasicum** – Foreign hospitals have used to treat gout/heart disease/high chol-BP. Clinical trials showed protect from cell mutation/bad bacteria/↑ blood to brain. (HSI)

- ➢ **Baking soda/lemon squeeze** – lowers uric acid levels w/1t in 8oz water/drink. Alkalizes acidity. 360 health

- ➢ **Raw organic apple cider vinegar** – 1 T in water/drink. alkalizes acidity. 360 health

Gray hair

- ➢ **Vit B$_5$** (Pantothenic acid) 100 mg + para-aminobenzoic acid (PABA) + 50 g brewer's yeast (3-6 months).

Gum Disease –3 x's increase in heart problems; 2 x's to have a stroke; worsen respiratory/bronchitis

- ➢ **Goldenseal/myrrh/calendula** Mouthwash. Make = 30 drop tincture each, add ¼ t to irrigator.

<u>Hearing loss/Tinnitus</u> – consider digestive test

➤ **Low HCL/pepsin**. IV inj. until digestion tests normal. Then, all oral. **Zinc & selenium** + all ess'l minerals + **Vit B$_{12}$ + B-complex** halts or reverses problem about 70%.
  - ✓ **Step 1**= digestion test/**digestive replacement therapy** of betaine hydro-chloride-pepsin or glutamic acid hydro-chloride-pepsin 1 cap/day (5,7 ½, or 10 grns) before meals 2-3 days. If no problems, 2 caps/day & cont. to gradually increase to 40-90/meal. Needs to be monitored by Dr (www.acam.org).
  - ✓ **Step 2** = 30 mg **zinc** 2 x's/day; 4 mg **copper** diff. times than zinc; 1000 mg **taurine** between meals; 800 IU **Vit E;** 300 mcg **selenium**; 80 mg **bilberry** 2 x's/day. Expect several months before any signs as needs to build up. (Dr Jonathan Wright)

➤ **Aldosterone** (+ potassium) studies show outperforming Prednisone® for age-related hearing loss 2005 study. Need to monitor electrolytes. www. canadaglobaldrugs.com & Key Pharm, www.keypharmacy.net. (Dr Wright)

➤ Too much **calcium**/too little **magnesium** = need 2 Ca: 1+ Mg (1000 CA/500-1000 Mg). **Vit D def.** or **B12** – check on this. Mixed results.

➤ **Foods to Avoid**: choc, dairy, bad fats, high salt. 360 Health

➤ **High omega-3** - associated with a significant reduction in the risk of age-related hearing loss (presbycusis) in people over the age of fifty. (Mercola)

➤ **Candida** – a common body fungal pathogen w/autoimmune hearing loss study (see Candida)

➤ **Vinpocetine** – see multi-symptomatic

➤ **Avena Sativa**– from wild oat plant & **Rosmarius Officinale** as nervous system tonic. 360 Health

➤ **Ginkgo biloba** w/24%flavone glycosides increases blood to brain… (Dr. Stengler - see more under cataracts)

Heart Disease/Stroke

– on auto-immune spectrum. Past 8 yrs = great paradigm shift to inflammation - **monitor homocysteine** levels especially if taking any drugs/supplements for cholesterol/diabetes. Never self-diagnose or treat. Do not mix meds w/supplements w/o Dr's OK. Also, electron beam computer tomography (artery-scanning tech) or plaque test = good indicators. U of Md Med Ctr = aspirin therapy ↑ risk coronary events in those w/healthy LDL. **Chronic inflammation =** underlying root cause for allergies/arthritis/psoriasis/diabetes/**heart disease/** cancer. See 'healing diets'. Also see *cholesterol* & *liver* sections.

➢ **Arjuna** – documented cure for ↓ LDL & overall chol + **angina** attacks (out performed ISMN). Also ↓ systolic BP & reduces BMI (wt. loss) also shown to correct atherosclerosis/ fight several types of cancer/ several types of E. coli/Salmonella infections. *"Arjuna – Cardiac Tonic"* (Himalaya USA)

➢ **CoQ$_{10}$** – considered the single most crucial compound for every cell in the body especially the heart but declines after age 25. 100-300 mg/day repairs **heart muscle damage,** ↓ cholesterol (LDL) & BP. CoQ$_{10}$ level test. *"CoQMelt"* = best delivery system (?) (under tongue) NorthStar Nut. (several sources)

➢ **Astaxanthin** – from H. pluvialis microalgae found in wild salmon – prevents oxidation/mutation of cells & ARMD, reduces inflam/**homocysteine**/LDL 26% w/NAC (JAMA/ Lancet/Nature/Heart Jl)/lowers cancer risks/**heart disease/** neurodegenerative diseases/stops cholesterol from oxidizing into plaque + Vit E (Harvard). www.astafactor.com. (Clark)

➢ **Nattokinase** (Fermented soybeans – Japan) de-clots blood (Dr. D Williams) & stim's production of clot-dissolving plasmin/ ↓ BP/combats senility/**prevents heart attacks**/strokes. 100 mg caps can replace Warfarin/**Coumadin**® (HSI)

➢ **Quercetin** - anti-oxidant found in broccoli/cruciferous vegetables reducing inflammation, healing 'leaky gut', calms immune system, targets atherosclerosis by reducing the "stickiness" of platelets, making them less likely to form into clumps that could obstruct fragile arteries. It also lowers harmful LDL cholesterol and helps to relax arteries, reducing stiffness and brittleness. (NH365)

➢ **Tocotrienols** – type of Vit E – dissolves arterial plaque+lowers chol/LDL. 200 – 400 IU/day. "***Care Diem***" = reduce/stop taking other drugs. "***PalmVitee***" (CompassionNet) – stops progression (92%), seen to reverse **atherosclerosis** (25%) (Dr Null +)

➢ **Chelation therapy** w/EDTA (AHA/FDA apprvd) - amino acid = heavy metals/dissolves **plaque**/improved joints/kidneys/inner ear/chol/atherosclerosis/↓ **homo-cysteine** levels/arthritis. "***Enhanced Oral Chelation***" caps = Vit's/Min's/Aminos. "2000 studies/100,000 satisfied users". (Health Res). Most common dose = 1-2,000 mg; "***Cardio Clear***" Health freedom Nut. www.hfn-usa.com. "***Metal Magic***" Baseline Nut. = removes 87% lead/91% mercury/74% Alum w/in 42 days

➢ **Hawthorn** – prevent/treat studies = recommended by German Commission - dilates coronary arteries/reduces BP/angina when taken over time/coronary artery disease/heart arrhythmia/congestive heart failure - by ↑ circulation/oxygenation to heart (underlying cause of angina). Has blood-thinning/diuretic effect. Enhances drug ***digitalis*** = more potent (↓ dosage), ↑ effectiveness of beta-blocker drugs/as effective as Catopril. 160-900 mg/day w/CoQ$_{10}$, Mg, L-carnitine. (Whitaker/Stengler)

➢ **Alcohol/coffee** – U of T study - protects brain from **stroke damage** if w/in 2 hrs - as eff as some ER drugs. (Williams)

➢ **Coffee fruit** – research show flavonoids ability to support heart health/strengthen vessels/uphold optimal metabolic processes/deliver oxygen to cells/support immunity/ anti-oxidants. (HSI)

➢ **D-Ribose** – 150 peer-reviewed published studies on how this carb is used in ATP energy production especially for heart function – return to normal in 2 days. (Weil+)

➢ **Zinc** – "quickest/easiest/effortless cure for **angina** in 14 days." Requires high doses of specific kind of Zinc. (Williams)

➢ **EPL** – supplement w/7 international studies document plaque melting away, angina gone, EKG's improve.

➢ **ALA** – clears oxidized LDL, blood vessels, dissolves plaque,…. see more in liver section.

➢ **Vit K** – deficiency linked to calcification/atherosclerosis; Increases cardiac/mitochondria output (foods–broccoli/kale/cabbage...)

➢ *"Cardio Vital Plus"* = ginger (thins)/motherwort (circ)/forskolin (art.)/**hawthorn** (strength)/**cayenne** (athero)/garlic (dissolves)/butcher's broom + willow bark (anti-inflam.)/bilberry (BP/eyes)/cordyceps (relax vessels)/mistletoe (BP/circ)/kelp (iodine). Biowell

➢ **Vit B_6/B_{12}/folic acid** – normalizes homocysteine levels - High levels = changes in artery wall/plaque build up + linked to **Alzheimer's**. *"Cardio-Support"* = 800 mcg EFA; 500 mcg B_{12}; 25 mcg B_6 (Adv Nut Pro.) Another study = 1 mg folate; 10 mg B_6; 4 mg B_{12}. (HSI+many)

➢ **Ginkgo Biloba** – terpene lactones - bioflavonoids/antioxidants prevent/treat as it increases circulation to brain, + **strokes**/cataracts/macular degeneration/diabetic retinopathy/**protects blood vessels**/lowers inflammation/relieves varicose veins, reverse **cardio-vascular disease**, & thins blood (↓ BP). 120-360 mg/day. Careful w/Coumadin/aspirin. (Dr Stengler)

➢ **Bromelain** – enzyme from pineapples aids in protein digestion (IBS), thins blood, breaks down **clots/plaques/angina**, anti-inflammatory (arthritis), varicose veins, thins mucus (CF or sinusitis), improves surgery recovery. 2,000 MCU/1,000 mg or 1,200 GDU/1,000 mg split into 500 mg 3x/day. (Stengler)

➢ **Nitric oxide** – proven effective by Mayo clinic to reduce cholesterol/**arterial plaque**/expands blood vessels (lowers BP)/controls platelet fcn/relieves impotency. Contains L-arginine + L-citrulline. (Bottomline Health) **"Enduracin"** wax-matrix for sustained release. (HSI)

➢ **L-carnitine** – helps transport fatty acids to heart for energy = **prevent heart disease**/high BP. 500-1,000 mg/day (Null). Taken w/in 24 hrs ↑ odds of **heart attach survival**. (Stengler)

➢ **Omega-3** fatty acids – calamarine/krill/algal sources decrease growth rate of atherosclerotic plaque + reduces risk of arrhythmias that lead to cardiac death. 3,000 mg/day. (Dr Null)

➢ **French Pine bark/pycnogenol + Gotu Cola** – works together to combat atherosclerosis/control plaque deposits. Pine bark/pycnogenol better than aspirin - breaks up plaque, stimulates production of nitric oxide, which prevents arterial constriction by helping arterial walls relax. Gotu kola helps inhibit plaque formation. NaturalHealth360/geenmedinfo.com

➢ **Pomegranate juice** – Proven study as antioxidant that removes/prevents **plaque**/reducing/reversing blood vessels damage & clears clogged arteries. 1 shot glass/day (Stengler)

➢ **Lecithin** – decreases melting point of hardened cholesterol when enough is present in blood. (Williams)

➢ **Cinnamon** - - helps w/metabolic syndrome (abdominal fat/blood sugar/BP. USDA study 1-6 g/day (1/4th – 1 tsp) for 40 days lowered glucose/ **triglycerides** by about 25% + **reduced LDL** up to 27%. (Dr Winston)

➢ **Cayenne pepper** (capsaicin) – a natural blood thinner helps **prevent heart attacks/strokes**. No Coumadin. Sprinkle on food/take in capsules regularly (Dr Null)

➢ **Larrea tridentate/Chaparral** = lignan NDGA – anti-oxidant/ anti-inflam/anti-viral/bacterial. Good after angioplasty. *Shegoi* LarreaRX, Inc www.shegoi.com.(HSI)

➢ **Nutritional Deficiencies** ; Vitamin C, vitamin E, beta-carotene, amino acids lysine, cysteine, arginine & proline; CoQ10, vitamin B-complex/folate, vitamin D3, MINERALS: calcium, potassium, magnesium, zinc, manganese, chromium, sodium, selenium, + carnitine, & pycnogenol. (Dr Rathe)

➢ **Prevention** –
  ➢ **Fiber** – 30-35 gm total fiber/day ↓ triglycerides, homo-cysteine/other markers. Flax seed meal sprinkle on food.
  ➢ **Foods**/herbs that reduce inflammation = walnuts, spinach, kale, all cruciferous/broccoli, probiotic foods like ACV & raw fermented veggies, onions, garlic, leafy greens, turmeric, rosemary, ginger.

> **Drinking tea daily** – Harvard study 44% lower risk of heart attack/lowers cholesterol, plaque buildup, & homocysteine levels. (Bottomline)

Heartburn/acid reflux – see ulcers

Heavy Metals/Toxicity/Poisoning –
causes inflammation in the body leading to other conditions Mineralpower.com. See detox as well

> **Chelation therapy** w/EDTA (AHA/FDA approved) - amino acid – clears out heavy metals/dissolves plaque calcium/ joints/kidneys/inner ear/cholesterol/ athero-sclerosis/↓ homocysteine levels/arthritis/kidney stones/ hearing loss. *"Enhanced Oral Chelation"* = Vit's/ Min's/Aminos. "2000 studies, 100,000 satisfied customers". Health Resource. Common dose = 1,000-2,000 mg. *"Cardio Clear"* Hlth Freedom Nut. **www.hfn-usa.com**; *"Metal Magic"* Baseline Nut'ls = removes 87% lead/91% mercury/74% aluminum w/in 42 days 800-695-5995. Rowen MD - **EDTA suppository Detxamin** = 36.3 % absorption rate over oral's 2-5%.

> **Chlorella/spirulina/cilantro/selenium/zinc/Vit C/ Glutathione** - help flush methyl-mercury from system. Jl of Toxicological Sciences reports results suggest that chlorella intake may induce the excretion of mercury. + Myersdetox.com

> **Foods:** garlic, onions, ginger, broccoli sprouts, egg yolks

> **Modified citrus pectin/grapefruit pectin** – attaches to heavy metals & eliminates them. MyersDetox.com

> **Binders**: most agree need to add a binder (taken away from food/supplements) to remove them from the body. Most agree best is clay (like zeolite/bentonite) or charcoal (many forms for cellular or intestinal; coconut charcoals) in nature. Seemingly & highly recommended by Dr Pompa/J Davidson is Systemic Formula's GCell & Bind products (2019).

Heavy Metals summary (Dr Fuchs)

Aluminum - absorbed & stored in the body is associated w/Alz-heimer's/nervous system & mental decline/behavior problems/ tooth decay/colds/constipation/energy loss/ hyperactivity/kidney problems/learning disabilities. To reduce risk, avoid it = anti-perspirants/aspirin/baking powder/cheese/pesticides/toothpaste/canned soft drinks…

Arsenic – known causes of brittle nails, diarrhea, nausea, convulsions, hair loss, headaches, lowered immunity, low-grade fever…. Best to avoid = insect sprays, pesticides, seafood (muscles/oysters/shrimp), rice,….

Cadmium – causes joint stiffness, pain/swelling, bone discomfort, liver problems, blood sugar imbalances, high cholesterol/blood pressure, impotence…. Best to avoid = candy, ceramics, fertilizers, fungicides, pesticides, evaporated milk, galvanized pipes, tobacco…

Copper – known causes of acne, allergies, anxiety, joint stiffness/swelling, reduced immunity, blood sugar imbalances, digestive problems, fungus, increased blood pressure/cholesterol, thyroid problems, migraines, bone loss, insomnia,… Best to avoid copper pipes, corn oil, ice makers, insecticides, liver, lobster, nuts, milk, soybeans, wheat germ, yeast,…

Lead – known cause of allergies, joint stiffness, back pain, vision problems, constipation, fatigue, headaches, blood pressure, reduced immunity, kidney problems, liver dysfunction, … Best to avoid = cosmetics, hair dyes, lead pipes, mascara, newsprint, pesticides, toothpaste, tobacco, wine,…

Mercury – known cause of brain damage, eye problems, emotional disturbances, dizziness, lowered immunity, joint discomfort, kidney problems, nerve fiber degeneration, numbness, vision loss,… Best to avoid = adhesives, air conditioning filters, body powders, cereals, cosmetics, dental fillings, insecticides, laxatives, pesticides, medications, soft contact lens solution, wood preservatives,…

Hemorrhoids – linked to dietary/dehydration

➤ **SSKI** – super saturated potassium iodide; *"TriQuench"* - 20 drps in 1 oz flaxseed oil applied.

➤ **Flaxseed** (ground) – added to food/drink + 300 mg **Butcher's broom**, 400 mg **horse chestnut** 15-20% aescin content 3X's/day (no herbs if on blood thinners) (Stengler)

➤ **Aloe vera gel** – applied; soothes/heals. 360 Health

> **Oak Bark** – cut 50 g into small chunks, boil 3 min/cool to warm. Pour into large basin & sit in it for 30 mins. 360 Health

> **Butcher's Broom** – Anti-inflammatory + ruscogen constricts veins/relieves swollen tissues. 360 health

Herpes outbreaks

> **Selenium** 250 mcg 2 x's/day + **lysine** 2 gms 2 x's/day between meals + **Vit C** 2000 mg 4 x's/ day + **Zinc** 30 mg 2 X's/day + **Vit A** 50,000 IU/day. "*HPX & HPX2*" BioTech Pharmacal

> *Oralmat* – Secale cereale extract liquid drops under tongue ↓/eliminates need for drugs + cold/flu/ viral/allergies/sinus.

> **Larrea tridentate/Chaparral** = lignan NDGA – anti-oxidant/anti-inflammatory/anti-viral/bacterial. Topical or supplement gives complete resolution to episodes w/in 24 hrs (replaces Acyclovir/Zovirax) + 90% pain relief for rheumatoid arthritis w/caps. for 2 wks. Good after angioplasty. *Shegoi* LarreaRX, Inc www.shegoi.com.(HSI)

> **Glycyrrhetinic acid ointment** – from licorice helps relieve painful sores/heal rapidly.

> **Beta-glucan** – originally for aqua-cultured fish farms. Based most ailments = micro-infections. By boosting immunity, many chronic, long-term ailments cured –arthritis/ chronic fatigue/HIV/herpes/cold/flu/allergies/ parasitic & bacterial infections. "*Immutol*" Immunocorp www.immunocorp.com)

> "**Viracea/Shing-Releev**" – successfully tested herbal treatment for **herpes/cold sores** & shingles. Stops spread of lesions, existing lesions begin to heal, & eases pain. Not if allergic to dandelions/aster family. (HSI)

> **Honey** - works better/faster than drugs for Herpes sores. Healing time with honey = 43% better than with drug for lip sores & 59% better for genital sores.

High Blood Pressure/Hypertension

Caused by damage to vessel's endothelial cells from toxins/A1C-sugar/insulin resistance/high fructose corn syrup = diet.

➤ **Magnesium Citrate** - Too much calcium/too little magnesium = most need to add **Mg** (500mg) – relaxes blood vessels. January 11, 2013 by Dave Mihalovic, '**Low Salt Diets Do Not Decrease Blood Pressure, Period.**' + '**The Salt Fix**' by DiNicolantonio - sugar as cause, selenium/Mg deficiencies.

➤ **CoQ10** – repairs heart muscle damage, reduces cholesterol/LDL/& BP. Can be taken w/meds 100-300 mg/day. www.BottomLineSecrets.com. "*CoQMelt*" best delivery system (?) (under tongue) NorthStar Nut'ls. 800-311-1950 (Wright)

➤ **Arjuna** – well-proven cure – Source CoQ10, reduces LDL/overall chol. + angina w/o side effects (better ISMN) + lowers BP, BMI (wt. loss) + correct atherosclerosis, fight several cancer types/E. coli/salmonella infections. 360 Health

➤ **Ginkgo Biloba** – terpene lactones -bioflavonoids/anti-oxidants prevent/treat Alzheimer's (apprvd treatment by German Gov.) as it ↑ brain circulation + strokes/protects blood vessels/decreases inflam/relieves varicose veins, reverse cardiovascular disease/**thins blood (↓ BP)**. 120-360 mg/day. Not w/Coumadin/aspirin. (Stengler)

➤ **Ginger** – 1 of most widely prescribed by Ayurvedic/Chinese for digestion disorders/arthritis/cardio-vascular disease/inflam/**thins blood (↓ BP)** - inhibits prostaglandin release (inflam.), enhances circulation, OK for pregnancy (1K mg max) not w/Coumadin; 250 – 2,000 mg (Dr Stengler)

➤ **Konjac mannan extract** – lowers BP/cholesterol + blocks fat absorption to help ↓ body mass index.

➤ **Omega 3s** – wild caught fish/krill/calamarine/algal sources.

➤ **Mouth Wash** – Dr Danenberg, 'if it kills bacteria, it reduces nitric oxide bacteria which can increase blood pressure'

➤ **Raw organic apple cider vinegar**–Drink 1 T in water 3x/day

➢ **Bromelain** – enzyme from pineapples - aids in protein digestion, thins blood (lowers BP), breaks down clots/ plaques, angina, anti-inflammatory (arthritis), varicose veins, & improves surgery recovery time. 2,000 MCU/ 1,000 mg or 1,200 GDU/ 1,000 mg split into 500 mg 3x/day. (Dr Stengler)

➢ **L-Arginine** – precursor to **nitric oxide** = blood vessel dilating metabolite to ↓ BP (Dr J Wright)

➢ **DHA/omega-3 fatty acids** – metabolite for ALA - 4 grams/day. (Dr. Jonathan Wright) Not fish - Krill/vegan

➢ **Forskohlin** – reduces pressure inside eyes, increases blood flow, + reduces blood pressure (Pres. Alt)

➢ **L-carnitine** – helps transport long-chained fatty acids to the heart for energy = prevents heart disease, high Blood Pressure, etc. 500-1,000 mg/day (Dr Null)

➢ **Dark Chocolate** – study in Hypertension, eating 3 oz/day = minor drops in BP/insulin resist/LDL chol. No sugar? = cocoa powder + Stevia or Lo Han

➢ **Berberine** – 27 double-blind, placebo-controlled trials shows = results to drugs for hypertension/BP drugs, high cholesterol (statins) and Type 2 diabetes (metformin) HSI/Mercola.

➢ **Lecithin** – 1 T /day liquefies arterial plaque (Dr. Williams)

➢ **Nutmeg** – a warming spice in Chinese med that brings blood out from center reducing over all pressure in body.

➢ **Potassium** 500+mg **+Ca** 1000 mg **+Mg** 500 mg (Dr J Wright) 100's of studies proving as effective as meds. Ask Dr. how much. John Hopkins – 33 different research projects. Best source Potassium = black-strap molasses.

➢ **Celery** - juice or 4 stalks/day = 3nB substance in oil w/ sedanolide & butyl phthalide relaxes blood vessels =lowers BP/blood flow/tumors in animals (NE La U School of Pharm & Univ of Chicago)

➢ **Black cumin seed oil** – one study, 1 tsp/day significantly reduced systolic measurements. (MGB)

➤ **Olive leaf extract** – out performs Captopril in lowering blood pressure + lowers LDL/triglycerides (J Landsman)

➤ **V-8 juice** – 13 different clinical trials + 1 study published in JAMA confirm lowers BP. (Dr Whitaker)

➤ **French maritime pink bark** - stimulates the production of beneficial nitric oxide, which prevents dangerous arterial constriction by helping arterial walls to dilate and relax.

➤ **Hot Cocoa** – stimulates production of **nitric oxide** boosting blood flow to heart/brain, etc. 1 study - thins blood as well as aspirin. Harvard professor claims treats blocked arteries, congestive heart failure, stroke, dementia, even impotence. 5 cups/day (Bottomline). Sugar problem? – make your own w/Stevia, xylitol, Lo Han (see diabetes) & nut milks.

➤ **Juniper Essential oil** – reduces BP in animal studies via anti-oxidants + natural diuretic, anti-cholinesterase slows heart, lowers BP/increase blood flow. Doctor's Harvest

➤ **Nutritional Deficiencies**: Vitamin C, vitamin E, beta-carotene, amino acids lysine & proline, magnesium, CoQ10, selenium, vitamin B-complex, folate, vitamin D3, calcium, potassium, zinc, manganese, chromium, carnitine, cysteine, arginine, Omega 3's, and pycnogenol. (Dr Rathe)

Foods:
➤ Any foods high in **vitamin C** (chili peppers, guavas, bell peppers, thyme, parsley, dark leafy greens, broccoli)
➤ Any foods high in **magnesium** (chocolate, green leafy vegetables, Brazil nuts, almonds, cashews, blackstrap molasses, pumpkin and squash seeds, pine nuts, black walnuts) + green coffee beans
➤ Any foods high in **potassium** (mushrooms, bananas, dark green leafy vegetables, sweet potatoes, oranges and dates).
➤ **Coconut** oil/water - very effective lowering blood pressure.
➤ **Most if not all spices** – not just ginger but turmeric/curcumin, clove, cinnamon, cayenne, even salsa

Note: do not eat or take these with blood pressure meds. Med's are taken away from food. Will find need less or no med's with these foods/supplements – Dr Nuzum.

IBS (Irritable Bowel Syn)**IBD/Crohn's/Colitis**

Caused by poor diet choices (refined/processed/fast foods), *stress*, food allergies/sensitivities (dairy/wheat/corn/soy/MSG/ artificial sweeteners), or genetic defect (Crohn's) that stim's immune response to bacteria. **Low FODMAP diet**

Dr. Lopez's 6-step program:
1. Remove all processed/refined foods/soft drinks/raw fruit replaced w/fresh, lightly cooked veggies for 2-3 wks.
2. Ban common food allergens (wheat/gluten/dairy/nuts).
3. Limit fluids while you eat.
4. Combinations of food can also cause problems. Don't eat potatoes w/protein & eat fruit alone.
5. Add a good digestive enzyme/HCL sup. (see below) to help protein digestion in the stomach.
6. Take steps to reduce stress.

➢ **Boswellia/Frankincense** – 200-400 mg 3 x's/day = 80% remission - out preformed Mesalazine® for **Colitis** & **Crohn's disease**. (don't take if have acid reflux) + add garlic, goldenseal, Echinacea & diet.

➢ **Digestive replacement therapy** of betaine hydrochloride-pepsin (HCL) or glutamic-acid hydrochloride-pepsin. See hearing loss for details (Dr J Wright+360 Health)

➢ **Probiotics: Fermented foods/Lactobacillus bacteria -** replace healthy bacteria in digestive tract. If SIBO, may aggravate. At health food store refrig section,… (potency questionable by how long in/out of frig.) – Kimchi,…

➢ **Blueberries** – Vit's/anti-oxidative/anti-microbial/fiber rich/polyphenols = reduce/protect against inflammation. Add Probiotics to increase effect. (Mercola)

➢ **Peppermint oil** – enteric-coated caps. 187 mg 3 x's/day or 1 drop oil in warm water, 15-30 min before meals ↓ abdominal pain/distension/stool freq./& flatulence.

➢ **Quercetin** – anti-oxidant found in broccoli/cruciferous vegetables reducing inflammation, healing 'leaky gut', calms immune responses, helps with IBS & Ulcerative Colitis.

➢ **Licorice Root** – Ayurvedic/Chinese med = harmonizing herb-detox liver/anti-inflammatory (stops prostaglandins)/boost viral interferon/**heals digestive tract (IBS/ulcers)**. High dosage can have side effects - sodium/water retention = ↑ BP, not if kidney problems/hypokalemia, not w/diuretics/digitalis. Tincture drops = 10-30 2-3x/day. Caps = 1,000 – 3,000 mg/day (Dr Stengler) – not w/kidney dysfunction

➢ **Aloe Vera** – 2 oz juice every 2 hrs relieves diarrhea, **colitis, IBS**, & boosts immunity. (several sources)

➢ **Sulfur** – homeopathic = cellular detox brings energy back when fatigued, + detox's digestive tract (ulcers/diarrhea/flatulence/**IBS**), relieves skin ailments (rashes/psoriasis/boils/eczema). Deficiency symptoms= always warm, sweats easily, no blankets, thirsty + likes sweet, spicy foods, fats, & beer. Other applications = headaches/insomnia/hot flashes/sore throat. 2 - 6C potency tabs 2/day for 2 weeks. For skin = may flare up temporarily due to detox. (Dr Stengler)

➢ **Ginger** – 1 of most widely prescribed by Ayurvedic/Chinese for **digestive disorders**/arthritis/cold/flu/vomiting/cardiovascular disease/stim's bile secretion/ reduces gas & bloating/thins blood (BP). It inhibits prosta-glandin release (inflame.),... OK for pregnant (1K mg max), **not w/Coumadin** + aggravates "warm-blooded". 250-2,000 mg (Stengler)

➢ **Turmeric/curcumin** in curry. Double-blind studies = reduces pain/stiffness from rheumatoid/osteo. + eases symptoms of **IBS/Crohn's**. 250-500 mg (std 80-90% curcumin) 3x/day. (Dr Wilson/Stengler)

➢ **Fiber/Prebiotic foods** – whole fruits/veggies for fiber + onion/garlic/inulin/chicory root,....bananas for diarrhea

➢ **Slippery Elm** - remedy for the symptoms of chronic GI problems such as leaky gut syndrome, ulcerative colitis, Crohn's disease, and irritable bowel syndrome. Dr Wm Cole

➢ **Peppermint Essential Oil** – anti-spasmodic/pain. 360 health

➢ **L-Glutamine** – (IBD/IBD/Celiac) heals gut lining by increasing size/height of villi, fuels immune cells. (Dr Osborne)

Immunity

- **Beta-glucan** – originally for aqua-cultured fish farms. Based on idea most ailments = microinfections. By boosting immunity, many chronic, long-term ailments gone – arthritis/ chronic fatigue/HIV/herpes/cold/ flu/allergies/parasitic & bacterial infections. *"Immutol"* Immunocorp 800-446-3063 x578B www.immunocorp.com)

- **AHCC extract** – Japan's medicinal mushrooms revs up *immune system*, destroys tumor cells, & prevents recurrence. Specifically, stimulates cytokine production, increases NK cell activity 300%, increases lymphocyte #'s/activity, interferon levels (lowers viral/bacterial infections), & increases formation of TNF proteins. 3 gm/day promotes **cancer** remission in trials. *"ImmPower"* (Harmony Co. 800-422-5518)

- *"ImmunoPhase/*Vital Cell formula."- Chinese broad-spectrum herbal prevent/treat **SARS/colds/flu.** Dr Dexin Yan's formula = Yin Chiao (1st signs of), Gan Mao Ling (decreases duration), Zhong Gan Ling (flu fever) + Pen Min Kan Wan (decongestant) + boosts immune = anti-viral/ bacterial/inflammation + decreases aches/pains. Can take any time to prevent. Tango Adv Nut 866-778-2646 (HSI)

- **Astragalus** – 500 mg/15 drops: herb curbs chronic **colds**, ear infections, & **flu,** has anti-viral/bacterial/ fungal prop's + prevent/treat cancer/protects against chemo damage/balance sugar & stimulates healing of kidney/nerve damage from high sugar levels/diabetes. **Boosts immune** fcn by increasing interferon & T-cells, macrophages, & NK, restores immune function in 90% of cancer patients & twice survival rate. (Stengler/Fuchs)

- **Bovine Colostrum** – immune-boosting = **"1st milk" w/antibodies**. (Dr Susan M Lark)

- **"Delta-immune"** – numerous Russia studies for long-term & immediate immune support - West Nile/colds/cough/ bronchitis/fatigue/hepatitis C/certain skin infections/yeast/ maybe cancer. Symptomatic relief is often w/in 12 hrs. (HSI)

➤ **Aloe Vera** – 2 oz juice every 2 hrs relieves diarrhea, colitis, IBS, & **boosts immunity**. (several sources)

➤ **Echinacea purpurea** – researched in Western Europe/US/ Canada w/clinical studies reinforce *immune boost* by increasing #/activity of phagocytes & antiviral chemicals = colds/ flu/sore throats/ coughs/toothaches. 500-1,000 mg every 2-3 hrs for acute; 2x/day for longer-term users. Should not be taken w/MS, tuberculosis, leucosis, collagenosis, AIDS, or other auto immune. (Dr Stengler)

➤ **Licorice Root** – Ayurvedic/Chinese med = harmonizing herb. Suppress cough/detox's liver/ balances hormones (PMS & menopause)/anti-inflammatory (stops prostaglandins)/boost viral interferon/chronic fatigue/heal digestive tract (IBS & ulcers). High dosage can have side effects - sodium/ water retention = increased BP, no for kidney problems/ hypokalenia, not w/diuretics/digitalis. Tincture drops = 10-30 2-3x/day. Caps = 1,000 – 3,000 mg/day (Dr Stengler).

➤ **N-acetyl cysteine** (NAC) – amino acid derivative/antioxidant that boosts immune function & has mucus-thinning prop's to help relieve wet cough w/phlegm & congestion in sinuses (cold/flu symptoms). 500-600 mg 3x/day (Dr Stengler)

➤ **Vit D** deficiency – linked to immune system. Dr. John Cannell, founder of the Vitamin D Council calls the flu a deficiency symptom. See multi-symptomatic section.

Incontinence/nocturia/nighttime urination
– can be due to allergies or other medical conditions.

➤ *"Bladder Tonic"* – liquid formula of 6 safe herb extracts for both males/females – lady's mantle/ partridge berry/gotu kola/St. John's Wart/witch hazel/corn silk. Wise Woman Herbals.

➤ **SagaPro Angelica** – herbal. Dr Teitelbaum

➤ For night time going, eat more dark berries (1 C/day) or 500 mg **quercetin** 2x/day w/meals, a strong antioxidant to decrease inflam/inhibits kidney cell damage. (Stengler)

Infections – bacterial/viral/fungal

If take antibiotics, add bromelain enzyme + after = probiotics. No willow bark for fever in children. No more antibiotics. See also Immunity. **Bacterial loves sugar/processed foods = avoid.**

➤ **Anti-microbials** (instead of antibiotics) summary: tea tree oil, oregano oil, garlic/allicin, biocidin, pau D'arco, cistus, ginger, turmeric, astragalus, Cat's claw.

➤ **AHCC extract** – Japanese medicinal mushrooms ↑ immunity = stimulates cytokine prod., ↑ NK cell activity 300%, ↑ lymphocyte #'s/activity, ↑ interferon levels (↓ viral/bacterial), & ↑ formation of TNF protein. 3 gm/day = cancer remission in trials. *"ImmPower"* (Harmony Co).

➤ *Colloidal silver* – UCI (Dr. Darryl See) testing on hard-to-kill *viruses & mycoplasmas family*, deep-seated micro-organisms (HSI) Dose 40-60 ppm. Compound pharmacies or Silver Edge Health/ Nutritionals has "micro-particle home colloidal silver generator" make own cheap. 800-528-0559

➤ *"ImmunoPhase/*Vital Cell formula."- Chinese herbal prevent/treat health workers - **SARS/colds/ flu.** Dr Dexin Yan's formula = Yin Chiao (1st signs of), Gan Mao Ling (↓ duration), Zhong Gan Ling (flu fever) + Pen Min Kan Wan (decongestant) + ↑ immune = anti-viral/ bact'l/ inflam + ↓ aches/pains. Can prevent. Tango Adv Nut 866-778-2646 (HSI)

➤ **"Bronchophase"** – blend 13 herbs dev by Dr. Fratkin for respiratory ailments/bronchitis. Published studies (HSI)

➤ *"Oralmat"* – Secale cereale ext drops under tongue reduces/ elim's need for drugs.Cold/flu/sinuses/allergies…. (several)

➤ *"Pain & Brain Rescue formula"* – *curcuminoids* from turmeric + *Boswellia* = anti-inflam. + *Gugulipid* = immune enhancer, anti-bact'l/viral/fungal, + *Bioerine* to absorb/use nutrients in food, better skin/energy. Inst. for Vibrant Living

➤ **Zinc** – for Alzheimer's/burns/**colds** (common ingredient in lozenges, "air-borne", Thera-Zinc spray) (Dr Stengler)

Infection – bacterial/viral/fungal, cont.

➢ **Olive leaf extract** - oleuropein, a potent antiviral, can stop the replication of cold, flu and shingles viruses (J Landman)

➢ **UBI therapy** – proven by several research centers for colds/ flu/pneumonia/hepatitis/strep/staph/blood poisoning/snake bites/tetanus/rabies/toxic mold/super-bugs quick. (Bowen)

➢ **Astragalus** – 500 mg/15 drops: herb curbs chronic **colds/**ear infections/**flu -** anti-viral/bact'l/fungal properties + prevent/ treat cancer/protects against chemo damage/stimulates healing of diabetes kidney/nerve damage. Boosts immune fcn by ↑ interferon/T-cells/macrophages/NK/restores immune fcn in 90% of cancer patients/doubles survival rate. (Stengler/Fuchs)

➢ **Aconie** – 1 of most common remedies for **flu/sore throat/ear infections/fever** - when symptoms come on fast after expose to cold/dry wind. 2 pellets 30C potency in mouth every 15 min for 1 hour only. (Stengler)

➢ **Echinacea purpurea** – researched in W Europe/US/Canada w/clinical studies reinforce immune boost by ↑ #/activity of phagocytes/antiviral chemicals = colds/flu/coughs/sore throats/toothaches. 500-1,000 mg every 2-3 hrs for acute; 2x/ day for no longer than 10 days. Should not be taken if have MS/TB /collagenosis/ragweed allergies/lupus/AIDS/any AI. (Stengler/Mars)

➢ **Ginger** – 1 of most widely prescribed by Ayurvedic/ Chinese for digestive disorders/arthritis/**cold/flu**/nausea/vomiting/ respiratory infections. Inhibits prostaglandin release (inflam.), enhances circulation, OK for pregnant (1K mg max) **not w/Coumadin** + aggravates "warm-blooded" people. 250 – 2,000 mg (Stengler)

➢ **Beta-glucan** – mushroom ext. Based on idea that most ailments = micro-infections. By boosting immunity, many chronic, long-term ailments gone – cold/flu/allergies/ parasitic & bacterial infections. "***Immutol***" Immunocorp 800-446-3063 x578B www.immunocorp.com)

➢ **Mullein** – herbal for ***coughs, chest congestion, mucus expectorate***, anti-inflammatory effects on respiratory tract. 30-40 drops 3-4x/day (Dr Stengler)

➢ **Tea tree oil** (Melaleuca alternifora oil) = anti-inflammatory/ analgesic/antiseptic/***anti-bacterial/fungal/viral*** for acne/ athlete's foot/boils/burns/cold sores/cuts/dandruff/ insect bites/lice/warts/ gingivitis (gargle)/vaginitis. 5% extract cream or gel; as a soap; or 10 drops-1 t in water (do not used undiluted). Not for infants. **Oregano Oil** has same affect - caps 500 mg 3x/day 8 wks. (Stengler)

➢ **Athlete's foot/Toenails –**
   ✓ Oregano oil/geranium oil/**tea tree oil** mixed 50:50 w/**DMSO** (transports it) rubbed over area daily for 1 wk (Athletes Foot) or 4-9 mos. (nails). (White).
   ✓ **Vinegar** – 2 drops base of nail 2x/day or soak in.
   ✓ **Tea tree oil** rubbed on nails 2x/day. (ICM)
   ✓ **Garlic** – steep 6 crushed cloves in a hot water basin for 1 hr & soak feet for 20 mins or ***allicidin/AlliMax***.
   ✓ **SSKI** – potassium iodide; topical for pimples/hangnails/ cold sores/toenail fungus (50 SSKI:50 DMSO mix) rub on.

➢ **Marjoram** – gargle for **sore throat**. Tastes bad. **Licorice/peppermint teas** – for **laryngitis + sore**

➢ **Anti-fungal formulation** = oregano oil + goldenseal + grapefruit seed ext + pau d'arco + probiotic + fish oil + fiber - rotated. (Dr Stengler). ***Allicidin/AlliMax (garlic)***

➢ **N-acetyl cysteine** (NAC) – amino acid derivative/antioxidant that boosts immune function & has mucus-thinning prop's to help relieve **wet cough w/phlegm** & **congestion in sinuses** (**cold/flu symptoms**). 500-600 mg 3x/day (Dr Stengler)

➢ **Vit D** deficiency – linked to immune system. Dr. John Cannell, founder of the Vitamin D Council calls the **flu** a deficiency symptom. See multi-symptomatic section

➢ **Green Tea extracts** – lab tests = stopped 3 different **flu** virus' from multiplying (Prev)

➢ **Bromelain** – an enzyme from pineapples that increases the effectiveness of antibiotics for every type if infection. 500 mg 4X/day. (Stengler)

➢ **Elderberry** extract - **Sambucol** 3 t/15ml 4x/day + garlic 500 mg 2x/day – study = reduces recovery time from **flu,** used less painkillers/fever reducers, & nasal spray.

➢ **Bovine Colostrum – *immune-boosting*** = "1ˢᵗ milk" w/antibodies. Dr Susan M Lark, MD

➢ **Hydrogen peroxide therapy** – into IV increases oxygen/cell activity/cytokines - own white blood cells (granulocytes) produce this to kill germs. (Campbell). **Cold/flu** – 3 drops in ear & bubble can cure in 12 hrs. (Mercola)

➢ **Cistus** - Plants in the *Cistus* genus exert a number of powerful antibacterial, antiviral, and antifungal properties against strep, staph, (prevent) ebola & HIV, candida, mold, & breaking down biofilms. (ProHealth)

➢ **Black Walnut** – liquid extract for **ringworm, athlete's foot, & jock itch.**

➢ **Cat's claw** – "..rids the body of infamous antibiotic resistant strep, which is frequently misdiagnosed as yeast/Candida. Strep is also true cause of many symptoms/conditions – **candida**/cystic acne/bacterial vaginosis/**SIBO**/sinus pain & congestion/otitis media/intestinal disorders/sore throats/ styes/**E.coli**/C. difficile/others; tremors, pain, + strengthens immune system to support **cancer**, ..." (medicalmedium.com)

➢ Sunlight/vit D (10,000 IU), **coconut oil**, turmeric, foods high in nicotinamide (vit B3 - salmon, sardines, nuts), + manuka honey, olive leaf extract, rose water, myrrh, onions, Oregon grapes, andrographis paniculate.

➢ **L-Glutamine** – amino acid that fuels immune cells + heals lining of the gut (leaky gut), some cancers, heals damage from chemo/radiation treatments.... Dr Osborne

Inflammation/Pain/Fibromyalgia –

Kenalog® = fake cortisone w/side effects. Ibuprofen/ Naproxen® = ↑ heart prob. (BMJ) + NSAIDs side effects = ulcers/bleeding/liver & kidney damage/osteoporosis/cartilage degeneration, leaky gut, etc. **Chronic inflammation =** underlying root to allergies/hormones/asthma/ arthritis/diabetes/osteo-porosis/heart disease/cancer = IL-6 test. **Linked to refined carbs, gluten, grains, sugar, bad fats (trans fats), GMOs, leaky gut, pesticides, heavy metals,…..**

➤ **"Flexagene"** - soothes aches/reduces swelling/repairs joints = contains **Vincara** (Uncaria guianensis ext.) turns down inflammation (Med Jl Inflam. Research) + RNI 249 (**Lepidium Meyenii** extract) stimulates/rebuilds joints & turns on gene responsible for producing IGF-1 (insulin-like growth factor 1) helps build lean muscle, burn fat stores, maintains skin, normalizes blood sugar. (Swiss Labs 800-619-7281)

➤ **Glucosamine/Chondroitin** – (glucosamine ↑ blood sugar; Chondrotin = no w/prostate + shellfish allergy) both = ↓ inflam/↑ lubricant/repair/rebuild. **"Flexanol"** (NorthStar) =G/C + MSM + **Boswellia +** EPA/DHA (omega-3 FA's)+ Borage oil & shell-fish free. If can't take – **Shark Cartilage –** same but natural. (several)

➤ **DMSO/MSM – DMSO** = liquid rubbed on w/cotton ball towards heart. Used for decades but recently approved by FDA – quick reduces inflammation/stiffness/pain. **MSM** (needs 50 mcg molybdenum supp if long term use) = caps/cream 2,000 mg/day. Can buy either straight or in **"Soothanol X2"** NorthStar Nut = DMSO + Emu oil + **MSM** + Arnica +… relief + rebuild. 800-311-1950

➤ **"Maxxima"** – 11 essential oils extracted from natural herbs. 25 European clinical trials/studies. Relieves pain, triggers body's healing mechanism to reduce inflammation., relaxes muscles. Biowell 800-877-2434

➤ **"Padma Basic"** – 19 Tibetan herbs for chronic leg pain due to intermittent claudication. 888-727-6388

➤ **Vit C, D, Folate, Magnesium** deficiencies – Dr Osborne

➢ **"Pain Erase"** - all natural liquid developed under Dr. John W Nelson, MD that "closes the gates of pain" left open even after healing has occurred. Erases arthritis/knee/migraines/ neuropathy/back/bursitis/hip/tendonitis/sciatica/neck pain for hours, sometimes days/wks/yrs. Harbor Health

➢ **Powerful Combo –**
  ✓ **Boswellia** – Indian herb 1000 mg ext. (400 mg boswellic acids)/day = ↓ inflam/ pain/ swelling/ increased flex./walking distance 90% in 1st 8 wks.
  ✓ **Willow bark ext** – "natural" aspirin (synthetic's origin) w/o side effects/more effective
  ✓ **Devil's claw** – (not if ulcers/preg./Coumadin) 1200-2500 mg/day aqueous ext. (also powdered = 5-10 g/day) for pain from So African plant - similar to ibuprofen/cortisone/outperformed Vioxx®. **Safe to take all 3** (White/Stengler)

➢ **"Pain & Brain Rescue formula"** –curcuminoids from **turmeric** + **Boswellia** (anti-inflammatory) & relieves arthritis, neutralizes metabolic wastes, **Gugulipid** converts excess cholesterol/burns fat/↑ levels of prostacyclin to zap abnormal platelets/detox major organs/↑ immunity, anti-bacterial/viral/ fungal/↓ stress, **Bioerine** to absorb/use nutrients in food, better skin/energy. Institute for Vibrant Living 800-218-1379

➢ **"TheraFlex"** = **Boswellia/Ashwagandha/Shatavari** for pain; **Bromelain/turmeric/& cinnamon** for inflam, **ginger/astaxanthin/rehmannia/licorice/ zinc/& copper** for detox/free radical eliminators; & **bioperine** ext (black pepper) ↑ bioavailibility. 800-270-4881

➢ **Mustard seed extract** (drops) stops joint pain, back strain, ankle sprains, golfer's elbow, & arthritis.

➢ **Turmeric/curcumin/ginger** – all detox & reduce inflammation. Take everyday 1000-3000 mg. (many)

➢ **Magnesium deficiency** – for muscle cramps, fibromyalgia, blood pressure, headaches, migraines, insomnia,… Best form is Magnesium glycinate. Avoid magnesium stearate (excipient)

➢ **"*Nexrutine*"** Phellodendron's yellow bark – berberine to make "super aspirin" (huang-po) w/o side effects – study shows relief of pain /inflammation/stiffness w/in 7 days. Solanova 800-200-0456

➢ **"*Lyprinol*"** An extract from green-lipped mussels-Eicosatetraenoic Acids (an Omega-3 FA) out performed Indo. for pain/inflammation but doesn't rebuild. Vitamin Shoppe 800-223-1216.

➢ **Bromelain** – 500mg 3x/day - enzyme from pineapple stems. ↓ inflammation/pain/swelling/& speeds healing. Or other proteolytic enzymes. Thins blood = not w/Coumadin®, fish oil, or Vit E. (several)

➢ **Protease** – enzyme that cuts inflammation/pain time 50% & improve healing time 50% as well. (Dr Null)

➢ **Fish oil/omega-3 EPA + DHA** – 1-1 ½ T/day or 500 – 1000 mg/day - reduces inflammation of arthritis, lubes platelets to ↓ cardiovascular problems. (several sources)

➢ **Bursitis = B$_{12}$ shots** – 2,000 mcg/day until pain is gone = best treatment for symptoms. Find cause = gastric/mineral/ folic acid (neurotrophilic hyper-segmentation index) analysis for low HCL – can't absorb B$_{12}$ supp/protein/minerals/ energy/ depression. Add HCL/pepsin capsules. (Dr J White)

➢ **Licorice Root** – Ayurvedic/Chinese med = harmonizing herb - anti-inflammatory (stops prostaglandins)/chronic fatigue/ heal digestive tract (IBS/ulcers). High dosage can have side effects - sodium/water retention = increases BP, not for kidney problems/hypokalenia, not w/diuretics/digitalis. Tincture drops = 10-30 2-3x/day. Caps = 1,000 – 3,000 mg/day (Stengler) – not w/kidney dysfunction

➢ **Ashwaganda** or "Indian Ginseng" – Ayurvedic remedy for fatigue/memory/asthma/bronchitis/psoriasis/arthritis/ stress/ anxiety/exhaustion/**inflammation/** anti-epileptic effect. Only few human studies so far. 1,000-3,000 mg/day (Dr Stengler)

➤ **Ginkgo Biloba** – terpene lactones -bioflavonoids/anti-oxidants prevent & treat Alzheimer's (apprvd treatment by German Gov. for effective delay of mental deterioration) as it increases circulation to the brain, + strokes, cataracts, macular degeneration, & diabetic retinopathy, protects blood vessels, reduces inflammation, relieves varicose veins, reverse cardio-vascular disease, & thins blood (lowers BP). 120-360 mg/day. Careful w/Coumadin/aspirin. (Dr Stengler)

➤ **Headaches** (also see migraines) – drink lemon balm tea (high in magnesium), add magnesium & fish oil sup. (omega-3s), avoid tyramine found in foods trigger vascular spasms – red wine/aged cheeses/deli meats/overripe bananas/MSG/nitrates/nitrites/all alcohol. (Magee)

➤ **Tendonitis** = DMSO + Vit E + trace minerals (liquid rub available from Tahoma Clinic Dispensary 800/893-6878 per Dr Wright)

➤ **Fibromyalgia** – chronic muscle pain + sore spots (tender points) = **ribose** 5 g powder 2x/day mixed w/water + **Mag** 250 mg2-3/day + **malic acid** 1,200 mg 2x/day + **CoQ$_{10}$** 200-300 mg/day improve w/in 2 wks (Stengler) **SAMe** + helps w/low energy characterized in fibromyalgia. 400-1200 mg/day. Not for Bipolar (HSI)

➤ **Foods/spices** that reduce inflammation = walnuts/spinach/kale/broccoli/rosemary/hot peppers/apples/onions/pineapples/flaxseed/olives-olive oil/cold water fish/berries/cayenne pepper/celery/celery seeds/cherries/dark green veggies – alkalizing .

Insomnia/dyssomnia (See also menopause)

➤ **Gotu Kola** – + good 4 agitation/anxiety/insomnia, epilepsy, hyperactivity (too much = rash+ sedation)

➤ **Valarian root** – (nature's Valium) (+**skullcap**) - ↑ serotonin brain levels, may contain GABA w/calming effect. As eff in tests as drug Serax w/o side effects. 300-500 mg 1 hr before bed. For kids 6-12 yrs = 160-320 mg VR + 80-160 mg **lemon balm** (German study in Phytomedicine) (Whitaker/Stengler)

- ➤ **Kava Kava** (good for stress too) – Hawaiian root. Don't take regularly/long term (over 30 days).

- ➤ **Melatonin** – levels rise during dark hours but may not be enough for some. 3 mg 1-2 hr before bed. (Stengler) Can increase dosage gradually to max 9 mg/day (Hauri)

- ➤ **Tryptophan** – 1000 mg w/water. Amino acid. (Whitaker)

- ➤ **Passionflower** – nerve relaxing properties for insomnia related to anxiety/stress; relaxes muscles, also good for hormone-balancing for PMS/menopause. 500-1,000 mg cap ½ hr before bed; 20-30 drops tincture; tea 2-3/day. (Dr Stengler)

- ➤ **Magnesium deficiency** – relaxes muscles, blood vessels,.

- ➤ **Sedalin** – combo of ziziphus spinosa + magnolia officinalis. Research proves works for 91% for insomnia - it regulates production of stress hormones, affects neurotransmitters in brain like meds, & calms central nervous system + slight antihistamine affect. (Stengler)

- ➤ **"Seditol"** – Magnolia -anti-anxiety/stress agents due to excess cortisol & zizyphus a traditional Chinese sleep inducer for over 2000 yrs. 365 mg nightly 1-2 weeks to notice changes. (HSI)

- ➤ **Inositol -** used for diabetic nerve pain, panic disorder, high cholesterol**, insomnia**, cancer, depression, schizophrenia, Alzheimer's disease, ADHD, autism, promoting hair growth, a skin disorder called psoriasis, and treating side effects of medical treatment with **lithium**

- ➤ **Linden flower/chamomile/passion flower teas**.

Kidneys/Stones (may be linked to oxalate issue)

- ➤ **Chanca Piedra** ext. Herb help expel/prevent (1999 study). Causes - dehydration/infection/Mg def./excess purines/Ca+ oxalates/uric acid = stones. 30 drops/day = 94% success. (HSI)

- ➤ **Magnesium citrate** – stones = Calcium oxalate. Makes Ca soluble. 500 mg/day. Add 50 mg B_6 = better results. (Stengler)

- ➤ **Baking soda therapy** – Dr Kopp solution reverses CKD 85%.

- ➢ **Astragalus** – 500 mg/15 drops: anti-microbial + stimulates healing of kidney/diabetic nerve damage. Boosts immune function by ↑ interferon/T-cells/macrophages/NK; restores immune function in 90% of cancers. (Stengler/Fuchs)

- ➢ **Malic acid** – found in fruit/apples dissolves stones.

- ➢ **Lemonade therapy** – Lemon juice is high in vitamin C helps dissolve stones. (Nutrition news) or high dose Vit C (many)

- ➢ **Foods**: red bell peppers/cabbage/ginger/onions/kale/spirulina/ chlorella/royal jelly/dandelion greens/cherries/berries/grapes/raw Apple cider vinegar/watermelon/parsley/cilantro/burdock/bone broth.

Liver/NAFLD (Fatty Liver Disease)/Stones

Primary detox organ/emotions, meds can cause problems (Statin's/ NSAID's/birth control pills/steroids), hepatitis, *toxic load* - heavy metals/*pesticides* (glyphosate)/fructose (HFCS)/diabetes/processed carbs/ nutritional deficiencies, sugar, EMFs,…. **ALT/AST/GGT blood test** = cell turn over or die off. Best score in low end of range. Liver issues show up as gallbladder, right shoulder/knee pain, …

- ➢ **Glutathione** (GSH) – a tripeptide; body's master antioxidant. Protects/boosts immune function/combats oxidative/ neuro-muscular diseases. Glyphosate disrupts production (glycine).

- ➢ **Betaine (HCl)** – amino acid in beets/spinach; breakdown of fats from liver + protect against toxins/chemicals/pesticides.

- ➢ **Alpha-lipoic acid (ALA)**. Check interactions. 600 - 1,200 mg/ day 4+ wks (many sources) *Dr Berkson's protocol:* - **ALA** 20 - 900 mg titrated + 20 mcg **selenium** + 2000 mg **milk thistle**/ day + binder (w/o food)/B's & Paleo or Keto-type/organic diet (see healing diets) regenerates/reverses Auto-Immune hepatitis.

- ➢ **Milk thistle** – used for over 2000 yrs to treat acute hepatitis, chronic liver disease, jaundice, chemical toxins/toxicity, & gallstones escorting toxins out of the body. (many)

- ➢ **Vit C** – high dose IV or oral ascorbic acid/sodium ascorbate powder (not pills); liposomal form to consider. < 50 gms (50,0000 mg)/day take to 'bowel tolerance' to flush system. Best in morning/home. Also helps *dissolve* stones. (several)

➤ **Cascara Sagrada** – laxative/colon cleansing/constipation + treats **gallstones, liver**, cancer. Was FDA approved for.

➤ **Foods:** walnuts (glutathione), carrots/juice (cleanse), leafy greens (chlorophyll bind toxins) - cilantro/spirulina/spinach/chlorella/spinach/kale, red apples (thins bile), bitters, radishes, peppermint, parsley, berries, clean water, cruciferous, dandelion root-greens/turmeric/Reishi mushrooms/gentian/garlic-onions (sulfur)/warm lemon water.

➤ **Others:** yellow dock root/probiotics/quercetin/olive leaf ext/berberine/oregano oil/Vit D, E, K/magnesium/ox bile/ zinc/phosphatidylcholine/resveratrol/Caster oil packs/green tea/carotenoids, Calcium D-Glucarate (CDG)/AMPK/TUDCA/DIM/fasting/Epson salt baths + binders (see detox) & exercise - all detoxes/thins bile/dissolves stones.

Menopause – no more "horse urine estrogen (HRT)!!" =
$\uparrow$ risk of cancer/heart disease/clots. Saliva test available for cortisol/DHEA/all 3 estrogens/progesterone/testosterone (+ thyroid check). Warning of deficiencies = autoimmune disorders/wt. gain/$\uparrow$ abdominal fat/depression/memory/hot flashes/hair loss/$\downarrow$ body temp.

➤ **Estriol** (E3) – Europe/Japan studies, w/estrone (E1) & estradiol (E2) as balance – Blood tests to estimate how much EQ = E3/ (E1+E2) + decreases cancer risks. Normal = 10% estrone/10% estradiol/**80% estriol**. www. aturopathic.org/ACMA

➤ **Progesterone cream/**oil drops) – bio-ID = precursor to other hormones + protects from osteoporosis. Dab wrists 2 wk/mo = physical/emotional/mental/sleep/stimulates bone growth (density up 15.4 - 30%)/thickens hair/restores libido/lowers fat/regulates thyroid/prevents cysts/vaginal dryness. (Williams) Health Resources. 20 mg cream 1-2x/day. (Stengler)

➤ **Pregnenolone** - hormonal balances of DHEA/progesterone/estrogen/testosterone + increases energy/mood/immunity/lowers rheumatoid/osteoarthritis/chronic joint/muscle pain/insomnia/cardiovascular/LDL/thyroid conversion of T4 to T3/cortisol/stress (**contains wheat**) (several sources)

➤ **Belladonna** – for throbbing hot flashes w/red facial flush along w/sweating. (Dr Stengler)

- ➤ **DHEA -** 5-15 mg/day– more important than estrogen for prevent/relieves hot flashes/other estrogen deficiency symptoms. Blood test for amount + check metabolites over time w/doctor (Dr J Wright)

- ➤ **"Estro-G 100"** – 3 herbal extracts = shanzhiside methyl etser, wilfoside, decursin/decrsinol work synergistically w/clinical results to relieve all common symptoms + acute/chronic joint pain & prevent osteoporosis (↑ bone density) w/o significant BMI changes or cholesterol levels but lower triglycerides. (HSI)

- ➤ **Sepia** – from cuttlefish ink. Treats hormone-related conditions = PMS/menopause/irregular cycles/ovarian cysts/fibro-cystic breast syndrome/bladder infections/ hypothyroid/low libido/ migraines/psoriasis/ sinusitis/meno-incontinence/uterine prolapse/vaginitis/ varicose veins. Stengler

- ➤ **Resveratrol** – Moravian red wine extract= French Paradox; anti-aging/↓ blood clots/bad cholesterol/plaque deposits/ balances hormones/anti-inflammatory/COX-2 inhibitor/ rejuvenates/immunity/corrects existing condition/diseases. Harvard/ Boston/Yale/No. Western…" (several)

- ➤ **Licorice Root** – Ayurvedic/Chinese med = harmonizing herb balances hormones (PMS/menopause)/anti-inflammatory (stops prostaglandins). High dosage can have side effects - sodium/water retention = ↑ BP, not for *kidney problems*/ hypokalenia, not w/diuretics/digitalis. Tincture drops = 10-30 2-3x/day. Caps = 1,000 – 3,000 mg/day (Stengler)

- ➤ **Passionflower** – good for hormone-balancing for PMS/ menopause + nerve relaxing properties = for insomnia related to anxiety & stress; relief, relaxes muscles. 500-1,000 mg cap ½ hr before bed; 20-30 drops tincture; tea 2-3/day. (Dr Stengler)

- ➤ **Gamma oryzanol** – compound in rice bran oil w/long history in Japan. 1 study = women w/hysterectomies 100 mg 3x/day for 40 days, 67% saw relief ½ of symptoms. 2nd study, peri-menopausal 300 mg for 4-8 wks, 90% improve, 40% excellent.

- ➤ **Vitex Agnus-Castus** – Relieves PMS & menopausal symptoms/balance hormones. Healthline.com

➢ **Maca** – HRT pre-gelatinized Peru only. Wt loss/decrease BP, hot flashes, cortisol, night sweats, depression, insomnia, anxiety, PCOS/increase pregnenolone, estriol, Fe, good HDL, iodine (thyroid). 2 – 500 mg caps 2x/day.

➢ **Natrum Muriaticum** – hot flashes + depression/insomnia that comes w/menopause. Other symptoms for this cure = craving salt. (Dr Stengler)

➢ **Cimifuga** – safe, 100's of years time-tested Native American herb. Studies effective for hot flashes/depression/ insomnia + may prevent cancer cells from metastasizing. (Stengler)

➢ **Wild Yam** – estrogenic effects when taken orally but suppresses progesterone syn. (Dr J White)

➢ **Black Cohosh/peppermint oil** - Hot flash/mood swings. Black Cohosh studies used at least 40-80 mg standardized to 2.5% triterpene glycosides (several sources)

➢ **Tribulus** – 500 -750 mg/day containing 45% steroidal saponins. Doesn't change hormones but relieves hot flashes/sweating/insomnia/depression. (Dr J White)

➢ **Boron** – USDA study finds women deficient – 2 apples & 1 handful of nuts/day = **3 more mg**/day doubled natural levels of most active estrogen causes decreasing symptoms, increased bone mass & sex drive. (Dr Inglis)

➢ **Shatavari root** – 1500 mg/day. Indian herb. Steroidal saponins increase desire. (Dr J White)

➢ **Sage+Alfalfa** - 1000-1500 mg. Clinical studies = hot flashes/ night sweating. (White) **Sage tea-**hot flashes/night sweats

➢ **Omega-3 fatty acids + Vit E** – 1 T Cod liver oil + 400 IU Vit E daily (Dr J Wright)

➢ **Cedar** - combo w/lavender rub into scalp = hair growth

➢ **Anthocyanins**: Reduces ovariectomy-induced learning and memory problems.

➢ **Blueberries**: Reduces ovariectomy-induced cellular aging (senescence) and bone loss.

➢ **Beans** (especially soybean) - Reduces ovariectomy-induced bone mineral loss.

➢ **Ginger -** Reduces ovariectomy-induced spatial memory loss.

➢ **Genistein** (in cultured soy, coffee, red clover): Superior to bone drugs Fosomax, Evista and Estradiol in reducing loss of bone strength and quality in ovariectomized animals.

➢ **Whey**: Reduces ovariectomy-induced bone loss in rats.

➢ **Coconut water**: Reduces ovariectomy-induced neuro-degeneration.

➢ **Plums/blackberries/black tea/EGCG (green tea)/ fennel**: Reduces postmenopausal and/or prevent ovariectomy-induced bone loss.

Migraines (neurological, vascular disease or genetic - triggered by environmental/mental (psychosomatic) or physiological factors/ causes or foods – wine/cheese/smoked fish/some beans/MSG/ meats w/nitrates/chocolate/citrus fruits/artificial sweeteners/ dairy/poor digestion/gluten/dehydration.

➢ **Procaine** – *"GH-3/H-3 Plus"* repairs damaged cell membranes to improve nutrient uptake 70%, ↓ % get diseases, lowers infections – help w/arthritis/cholesterol/**migraines**/ heart/MS. Covered on 60 min – 100 mil people use. *"Ultra H-3"* 1-2 x/day Uni Key Health Sys. www.unikeyhealth.com.

➢ *"Pain Erase"* - all natural liquid developed under Dr. John W Nelson, MD that "closes the gates of pain" left open even after healing has occurred. Erases pain from arthritis/knee/ **migraines**/neuropathy/back/ bursitis/ hip/tendonitis/ sciatica/neck/& headache for hours, sometimes days, weeks, or even years. Harbor Health 888-859-9800

➢ **Feverfew** – clinical studies show prevents a migraine headache before it hits/reduce severity. "**MigraSpray**" – 4 traditional homeo herbs: feverfew/goldenseal/ dandelion/polyporus officinalis – contributes factors adding to anti-inflam feverfew. MigraSpray says no preg/lactating/blood-thinners/NSAIDs. 10 sprays under tongue. (HSI+)

- ➤ **Butterbur extract/Petadolex** – 50-75 mg 2x/day = 50% fewer migraines prevents blood vessel inflam.

- ➤ **Prevent migraines/headaches** w/200 mg Magnesium glycinate + 500 mg Calcium citrate 2x/day (Stengler).

- ➤ **Magnesium/Vit B$_6$** inj = inexpensive if do it yourself.

- ➤ **Vit B$_2$** (riboflavin) – 400 mg/day reduces # & severity.

- ➤ **Headaches** – drink lemon balm tea (high in magnesium), add magnesium & fish oil/omega-3s & avoid tyramine found in aged/fermented foods trigger vascular spasms – red wine/aged cheeses/deli meats/overripe bananas/MSG/nitrates/nitrites/all alcohol. (Magee) + no soda.

Morning Sickness/nausea/motion sickness

- ➤ **"Vertigoheel"** – homeopathic remedy w/cocculus from cockle plant to relieve dizziness/vertigo/motion sickness. (Dr Lengyel)

- ➤ **Ipecac** – a homeopathic remedy works on all kinds of nausea in as little as 5 mins. (Stengler)

- ➤ **Vit K** 5 mg + Vit C 250mg + Vit B$_6$ 25 mg + **ginger** 125 mg 2-3x/day

- ➤ **Ginger** – candy/ale/teas/caps for **nausea.** 1 of most widely prescribed by Ayurvedic/Chinese for digestive disorders/flu/cold/nausea/**vomiting**/motion & **morning sickness**/thins blood (BP). Inhibits prostaglandin release (inflam), enhances circ, OK for pregnant (**1K mg max**) not w/Coumadin + aggravates "warm-blooded" people. 250 – 2,000 mg (Stengler)

- ➤ **Marshmallow** (Althaea off.) **or licorice root** (glycyrrhiza glabra) **extracts** – speed recovery from intestinal flu, ulcers, food poisoning.

Multiple Sclerosis (MS) – Research in England has linked 61% to **Vit D** deficiency + glandular fever – total 71% cause (BBC/Mercola). Also listed under possible psycho-somatic origin. (Dr Sarno "The Divided Mind") & low-grade infections (candida).

➢ **Procarin** – amino acid derivative – a histamine that may restore blood flow to affected tissue – 67% = at least 1 or more significant improvements. Available in skin patch by prescription from compound pharmacy.

➢ **Procaine** – *"GH-3/H-3 Plus"* repairs aged/damaged cell membranes to improve nutrient uptake 70%, reduces % get diseases, reduces infections – help w/arthritis/depression/ emphysema/heart disease/Hodgkin's/**MS**/migraines/ osteoporosis/ Parkinson's. Covered on 60 min – 100 mil people use. *"Ultra H-3"* 1-2 x/day www.unikeyhealth.com.

➢ **Calcium aminoethylphosphate** (CaAEP) injectable (Dr. Hans Nieper of Germany) - improvement in majority of patients in 13 of 36 possible sym.

➢ **B_{12} Deficiency/injections** 1-2x/wk + sublingual daily – prevent/treat flare-ups + **fish oil/cod liver oil EFA** + **evening primrose** GLA + **Vit D** (Dr Stengler) + restrictive diet (=Dr Swank of U of O Med School) halts progression.

➢ **Dr Wahl's protocol** – a dietary approach where she reversed her MS using foods, detox, stress reduction – a no-grain, organic, Paleo diet protocol high in 31 brain nutrients of 3 C leafy greens/3 C colored veg/3 C sulfur-rich veg/…..

➢ **Vit D** – deficiency link. Tests: MCH/homocysteine/MMA. (Dr Osborne) – he also mentions **Biotic** deficiency.

➢ **Lion's Mane** – NGF/stim's myelination of nerves.

➢ **Niacin deficiency** – No-flush 2000 mg/day reversed MS & Dementia. (Dr Ben Johnson)

➢ For **MS muscle cramps – magnesium cream/oil** or DMSO + Magnesium in transdermal cream (prescription) Key Pharm. 800-878-1322 www.keynutritionrx.com (several sources) + Vit K

Muscle cramps/spasms — repetitive = mineral deficiency or digestive problem if over 40.

➤ **Potassium/Mag/Cal/Vit E** (tocopherols)/**Vit K** supplements.

➤ For MS or CP – **magnesium cream/oil** or DMSO + Mg in a transdermal cream (prescription.) Magnesium cream rubbed on will relax nerves/muscles. (Dr Stengler) Key Pharmacy 800-878-1322 www.keynutritionrx.com

➤ **Ignatia** – for depression brought on by grief or disappointment, stress/tension headaches, **muscle tension**, & PMS. Many practitioners (psychologists & counselors) have observed quicker recoveries/ dramatic changes in outlook. 30C 2/day for a week (Dr Stengler)

➤ **Gastric analysis test. Low HCl/pepsin.** IV inj. until digestion tests normal. Then, all oral. **Zinc & selenium** + all ess'l minerals + **Vit B$_{12}$ + B-complex** halts or reverses problem about 70%.

  ✓ **Step 1**= digestion test/**digestive replacement therapy** of betaine HCl-pepsin or glutamic acid hydro-chloride-pepsin 1 cap/day (5,7 ½, or 10 grns) before meals 2-3 days. If no problems, 2 caps/day & cont. to gradually ↑ to 40-90/meal. Needs to be monitored by Dr (www.acam.org).
  ✓ **Step 2** = 30 mg zinc 2 x's/day; 4 mg **copper** diff. times than zinc; 1000 mg **taurine** between meals; 800 IU **Vit E;** 300 mcg **selenium**; 80 mg **bilberry** 2 x's/day. Expect several months before any signs as needs to build up. (Dr Jonathan Wright)

➤ **Indium** – see multi-symptomatic

Osteoporosis – urine test = measures breakdown + DEXA X-ray baseline age 50, then 1 x/3-5 yrs.

Maybe due to **too much** Ca or P (decalcifies), or too little Mg (to absorb Ca), **Vit D, Vit K, EFAs, Boron**, Strontium (taken separately), or Silicon all needed. **Chronic inflammation** = underlying root to allergies/asthma/arthritis/psoriasis/diabetes/**osteoporosis**/heart disease/cancer = **IL-6 test.** Milk can raise fracture risk by 45% as triggers inflammation.

➤ **Progesterone cream** – precursor to other hormones + stimulates bone-building to protect against osteoporosis. Dab on wrists 2 wk/mo = physical/ emotional/ mental/ stimulates bone density ↑ 15.4 -30% + thickens hair/restores libido/↓ fat/regulates thyroid. (Williams) Health Resources 800-471-4007/ most health food stores carry plant-identical.

➤ **Procaine** – *"GH-3/H-3 Plus"* repairs aged/damaged cell membrane to improve nutrient uptake 70%, reduces % get diseases/ infections – help w/acne/arthritis/ depression/ emphysema/ cholesterol/heart disease/ Hodgkin's/migraines/MS/**osteoporosis**/Parkinson's. Covered on 60 min – 100 mil people use. *"Ultra H-3"* 1-2 x/day Uni Key Health Sys. www.unikeyhealth.com.

➤ **Ipriflavone** - increases osteoblasts/reduces osteoclasts activity by raising hormone responsible = maintains/ increases bone density w/o estrogenic effect. 60+ Clinical studies over 10-15 years have been positive when w/Ca, Mg, Vit D, Zn, Ma, C, B_6, B_{12}, boron,, K, ... 200 mg/3 x's/day w/meals. No if kidney disease + watch lymphocyte levels. (Dr Stengler)

➤ **"Estro-G 100"** – 3 herbal ext = shanzhiside methyl etser, wilfoside, decursin/decrsinol work synergistically w/clinical results to relieve all common symptoms + acute/chronic joint pain & prev osteoporosis (↑ bone density) w/o significant BMI changes or cholesterol levels but lower triglycerides. (HSI)

➤ **cumin seeds** - capable of inhibiting loss of bone density and strength as well as hormone therapies in women. www.greenmedinfo.com

➢ **Calcium/magnesium ratio** = need **2 Ca: 1+ Mg** (1000 CA/500 Mg). Add **Strontium** supp. prevent/ treat. (Fuchs). Too much phosphorus (Williams)

➢ **"Osteoking"** – **A**stragalus root, Asia Gingeng root, safflower, Tienchi Gingeng root, Eucommia bark, tangerine peel can actually heal **bone fractures** in as little as 3 wks based on kidneys converting calcitriol to Vit D. Many restrictions (HSI)

➢ **Potassium Citrate** – boosts bone density in post- menopausal (alkalinity). Jl Am Society of Nephrology. 30 mg/day

➢ **"OsteOrganiCal"** – in 300 separate treatment studies, ↑ bone mass by 3% in 3-6 months, 18% in 15 months, w/a maintenance program of 2-3 mo/year based on coastal algae content of Ca/Vit D_3. Natural options Corp 800-516-9796

➢ **DHEA -** (5-15 mg/day)– more important than estrogen to prev osteoporosis/relieves hot flashes/estrogen deficiency symptoms. Blood test amount/check metabolites over time (Wright)

➢ **"Osteophase"** – made from oyster shell lining combined w/21 diff amino acids, iron, zinc, & 3 herbs – Astragalus/Angelica sinensis root/Coix seeds that reduces Ca loss/↑ bone density & remodeling by reliably regulating Ca homeostasis.

➢ **Sesame seed oil** = 1 way to get Ca. Chinese cook w/it, avoid milk/cheese, & still have stronger bones (Dr Null) + get enough Mg /Vit D (Dr Stengler).

➢ **Boron** – USDA study finds women deficient – 2 apples & 1 handful of nuts/day = **3 more mg**/day doubled natural levels of most active estrogen causes decreasing symptoms, increased bone mass. (Dr Inglis) See 'the boron conspiracy' paper.

➢ **Rosemary -** specifically phyto*cannabinoid* is beta-caryophyllene or BCP has shown to promote bone formation/mineralization, which may prevent osteoporosis. MBG blog.

➢ **Foods**: Dates, figs, prunes, apples, berries, pears, grapes, pomegranates.

> **Butter/butter extract** – richest source of factor X bone building nutrient. (Williams)

> **Eat more alkaline foods** = leafy veggies/squashes/pears/ bananas/melons/brown rice. (Dr Stengler) **Prunes** – eating them shown to build stronger bones (Bottomline Health)

Parkinson's

– auto-immune spectrum. New studies show can be due to excess manganese (toxicity) & does not respond to Levodopa drug. Also linked to leaky gut/leaky brain/candida/high blood sugar/gluten/ lack of *Prevotellaceae family bacteria*. See **AIP/Keto** in 'healing diets'.

> **Manganese-induced Parkinson's toxicity -** exposure to steel manufacturing/welding/gas = para amino salicylic acid (PAS). So far, 80 people treated successfully/permanently. (Rowen MD)

> **Glutathione** (GSH) – a tripeptide of cysteine/glutamine & glycine offers antioxidant protection, reverse fatigue, superior immune function, & detox to combat oxidative/neuro-muscular diseases. GHS precursor, cysteine, derived from milk whey is body's preferred form used to treat Parkinson's + strong antiviral. 500 mg/day *CysteinePeP* NutriCology 800-545-9960 www. nutricology.com (+ 1,000 mg vit C & n-acetylcysteine 500 mg 2x/day + 300 mg ALA Dr Stengler)

> **Lion's Mane** – Stim's NGF/nerve regeneration/plaque.

> **Procaine** – "*GH-3/H-3 Plus"* repairs age/damaged cell membranes to improve nutrient uptake 70%, reduces % get diseases/infections – help w/arthritis/depression/heart disease/MS/**Parkinson's**. Covered on 60 min – 100 mil people use. "*Ultra H-3"* 1-2 x/day www.unikeyhealth.com.

> **CoQ$_{10}$-** Enzyme for energy & heart now confirmed in clinical trials by Nat'l Institute of Health w/higher doses to help Parkinson's patients. (Dr Whitaker)

> **Vit K deficiency** – neuroprotective, increase function; linked to calcification/athero; Increases cardiac/mitochondria output (foods – broccoli/kale/cabbage….)

> **Fluoride -** neurotoxin that calcifies in the brain. Filter water.

PMS – oral contraceptives study in Am Jl of Obstetrics/Gyno = 37% decrease in CoQ_{10} & 23% alpha-tocophenerol levels + deplete body of nutrients (B's/Mg/Zn/Vit C). Need to add extra + possible iron deficiency – simple blood serum test.

➢ **Omega-3 oils** (fish/flax seed oils) 1 T/day (1000 mg) = reduces cholesterol/heart disease/rheumatoid arthritis/joint pain/ breast cancer/asthma/diabetes/insulin resistance/ menstrual cramps/**PMS**/psoriasis/eczema/stroke/flaky skin/ split-brittle nails/"bumpies" on back of arms. (several)

➢ **Evening Primrose Oil** = omega-6 EFA/GLA – PMS/cyclic breast pain/eczema/diabetic neuropathy/arthritis pain. GLA = inflammation, prevent clots/reduce cramping/ balance hormones/prevent nerve damage from diabetes. For Eczema/ **PMS** = 150-400 mg GLA (1,500-3,000mg oil) + omega-3 oil supplement taken w/meals. (Dr Stengler)

➢ **Licorice Root** – Ayurvedic/Chinese med = harmonizing herb that **balances hormones** (**PMS** & menopause)/anti-inflam-matory (stops prostaglandins)/boost viral interferon. High dosage can have side effects sodium/water retention = increases BP, not for kidney problems/hypokalenia, not w/diuretics/ digitalis. Tincture drops = 10-30 2-3x/day. Caps = 1,000 – 3,000 mg/day (Dr Stengler)

➢ **Ignatia** – for depression brought on by grief or disappointment, stress/tension headaches, muscle tension, & **PMS**. Many practitioners (psychologists & counselors) have observed quicker recoveries/ dramatic changes in outlook. 30C 2/day for a week (Dr Stengler)

➢ **Passionflower** – nerve relaxing properties = for insomnia related to anxiety/stress; relief, relaxes muscles, also good for hormone-balancing for PMS/menopause. 500-1,000 mg cap ½ hr before bed; 20-30 drops tincture; tea 2-3/day. (Stengler)

➢ **Krill oil** (omega-3 FA) – studies show for **PMS, cramps**, inflammation better than fish oil. 2 g/day. Blood-thinning effect so no Coumadin. (Dr Stengler)

<u>Prostate</u> – 50% of all men = problems. Elevated PSA test only related to prostate size, not cause. 2/16 ratio (2.0 or better) – 2/16 home testing kits available by mail. Aromatization process turns testosterone into estrogen = ↑ risk. Check it. Can also be caused by too much Ca/ not enough Mg/Vit D or "prostate congestion".

➢ **Stinging nettles** – works better than others alone. Add **Saw palmetto** &/or **Pygeum** & they become just as effective as any drug w/fewer side effects. (Stingler) **"Prostate Defense"** = **Saw palmetto** – Serenoa Repens (sterols) + **Stinging needles** – Urtica Doica + **Pumpkin seed** – phytosterols + **Pygeum Africanum** (bark). North Star Nut'ls 800-311-1950; **"Prostate Essentials Plus"** – Swanson's; **"Herbal Prostate Combo"** or **"Saw Palmetto Combo"** has 3 or 4 of above (higher dosages) www.swasonvitamins.com

➢ **Testosterone deficiency** = heart disease/prostate/depression/ cholesterol/abdominal fat. Studies show marked decreases in all parameters measured. Have PSA checked before & after 3 mos. 80-120 mg Androderm & Testoderm TTS patches, creams/gels cheaper, or oral from compounding pharmacy. (Wright)

➢ **Ubiquinone** – CoQ 10-enzyme decreases w/age = deterioration tied to heart/baldness/wrinkles/ eyesight/hearing/gums/arthritis/age spots/bladder control/**prostate**. Noble prize winner Dr P Mitchell, Dr Wm V Judy, AMA/JIM/JN/US Gov NIH/ UCLA Med School/ Indiana Univ Med school. "**Ubitol**" – BioNutrigenics, 800-206-9872)/ "**Cardigen**" – Swiss labs, 800-301-9471)

➢ **Lycopene** – found in tomatoes/watermelon + Zinc – 90 mg chelated + Selenium – yeast + copper - 2 mg, Vit E – 400 IU (alpha/beta/gamma tocopherols) + **Fish oil** (distilled) or **flax oil** – 2T (EFA deficiency). Eat more fish – mackerel, salmon (wild), catfish, flounder, perch, sole, & cod (careful of mercury), unroasted sunflower seeds. Can add **Maitake** or **Coriolus versicolor** medicinal mushroom extracts + **astragalus** root to boost immune responses. (several)

➢ **Selenium** – 200 -300 mcg + 20 -30 mg **lycopene**, + 3 mg **boron** = further protection (Dr. J Wright)

➤ **Beta Sitsterol** – plant fat shown in major studies published in British Jl of Urology/Lancet to boost urine flow/empty bladder & more affordable than others. (Campbell)

➤ **Crinum lactofolium** – traditional Vietnamese medicine. 7 yrs of research/500 case histories = 92.6% success for BPH symptoms – not yet confirmed US studies. (HSI)

➤ **Brassicca veggie** (mustard family) + 1 T fresh ground flaxseed/day; **DIM** supplement to balance hormones 60 mg 3x/day & recheck 2/16 after 4-6 wks. **Chrysin w/diadzein** – from **passionflower**. If aromatization excess, 500 mg 3x/day. Re-check in 4-6 wks (Dr. J Wright)

➤ **Zinc** – long-term use depletes body of copper. 90 mg/day for 2 months, 50 mg/day maintenance after. (Stengler)

➤ **Pomegranate juice** – 1 shot daily serving slowed division of prostate cancer cells (HSI)

Psoriasis/Shingles – allergy related? Do full sensitivity tests (see allergies). (Wright) **Chronic inflam =** underlying root cause.

➤ **Mahonia Aquifolium** – 10% extract from Oregon grape = success w/1000s – 81% improvement in 12 wks. Inhibits proliferation of skin cells, ↓ inflam., & anti-bacterial/fungal. *M-Folia* NorthStar Nut. www.northstarnutritionals.com.

➤ **Burdock** – eczema/acne/**psoriasis/**chronic urinary tract inf. Detox = supports liver/destroys blood im-purities (bacteria/yeast), improves lymphatic system/ dig./elim. Rich in minerals, phytonutrients, & stim's metabolism/healing. 300-500 mg 2-3/day (Dr Stengler)

➤ **Sulfur** – homeopathic = cellular detox brings energy back when fatigued, detox's dig tract, relieves skin ailments (rashes/ **psoriasis**/boils/eczema). Deficiency symptoms = always warm, sweats easily, no blankets, thirsty + likes sweet, spicy foods, fats, & beer. Other applications = headaches/insomnia/ hot flashes/sore throat. 2 - 6C potency tabs 2/day for 2 wks. For skin = may flare up temp due to detox. (Dr Stengler)

- ➤ **Ashwaganda** or "Indian Ginseng". 1000s of years Ayurvedic remedy for fatigue, impotency, memory, asthma, bronchitis, **psoriasis**, arthritis, stress, anxiety, exhaustion, inflammation. few human studies. 1,000-3,000 mg/day (Dr Stengler)

- ➤ **Tamanu oil/Calophyllum inophyllum** – effective cicatrizing agent w/anti-bact'l/inflam & antioxidant prop's. Calophyllic acid is unique fatty acid here + xanthones + coumarins. Used topically for eczema/**psoriasis/shingles**/ rheumatism/neuralgia/ wounds/ blemishes/wrinkles. (HSI)

- ➤ **"Viracea/Shing-Releev "** – successfully tested herbal treatment for herpes/cold sores & **shingles**. Stops spread of lesions/heals existing lesions/eases pain. (HSI)

- ➤ **"Shingles Relief"** – anti-neuralgic/viral herbs/com-pounds = humic acid/poke root/chaparral/lemon balm (type 1 & 2)/ white willow bark/arnica/meadowsweet/comfrey/aloe vera = relief from pain/nerves. Nature's rite. (HSI)

- ➤ **Geranium oil** – 100% geranium oil. Study group experienced greatest pain relief from **shingles**' post-herpatic pain. Some experienced slight skin irritation/less w/50/50 solution. (HSI)

- ➤ **Nickel + bromide prep** - www.lomalux.com (HSI)

- ➤ **1.25 dihydroxy Vit D** (through compound phar-macies) + 1000-3000 mcg **Vit B₁₂** + 50 mg **folic acid**

- ➤ **Forskolin** – 5 mg 2-3 x's/day. Ayurvedic medicine.

- ➤ **Fumaric acid** – cells don't produce enough of this & start producing chemicals that irritate skin. Many clinical studies show 4 out of 5 patients saw dramatic relief w/supple-mentation + dietary changes. Minor tingling or flushing sensation for side effects (Br J Dermatology 05/Williams)

- ➤ **Inositol** is used for diabetic nerve pain, panic disorder, high cholesterol, **insomnia**, cancer, depression, schizophrenia, Alzheimer's disease, ADHD, autism, promoting hair growth, a skin disorder called psoriasis, and treating side effects of medical treatment with **lithium**

Restless Leg Syndrome

Restless Leg Syndrome – assoc dialysis/iron-mg-folic acid deficiency/heavy smoking/obesity/snoring/hypertension/ anti-depressants/diabetes/lack of exercise/circulation.

➢ **Valerian** (nature's valium), **skullcap, & passion-flower** – good for nervous system & sleep.

➢ **Calcium** Citrate or chelated + 250-500 mg Magnesium every night. Check deficiencies in iron/folic acid/Magnesium. Check low blood sugar = protein bar at night. (Stengler)

➢ **Horse chestnut** 2.4 g/**butcher broom** 1.6 g/**ginkgo biloba** 4-6 g (80-120 mg of std 50:1 extract) – ↑circulation.

Rosacea

Rosacea – Assoc. w/↓ stomach acid = gastric analysis test. If stomach, replacement therapy = Low HCL/pepsin. IV inj. until digestion tests normal. Then, oral. Zinc/selenium + all essential minerals+Vit B_{12} + B-complex halts or reverses problem about 70%.

✓ **Step 1**= digestion test/**digestive replacement therapy** of betaine hydro-chloride-pepsin 1 cap/day (5,7 ½, or 10 grns) before meals 2-3 days. If no problems, 2 caps/day & cont. to gradually up to 40-90/ meal. Needs monitoring by Dr (www.acam.org).

✓ **Step 2** = 30 mg **zinc** 2 x's/day; 4 mg **copper** diff. times than zinc; 1000 mg **taurine** between meals; 800 IU **Vit E;** 300 mcg **selenium**; 80 mg **bilberry** 2 x's/day. Expect several months before any signs as needs to build up. (Dr J Wright) HCL + pepsin + Vit B_{12} /B complex

➢ Or **Helicobacter pylori** – bacterial infection – get test (see ulcers)

Smoking

➢ **Plantago Major/Broadleaf plantain** – commonly used for bronchitis/lung ailments + natural aversion to tobacco eliminating pleasure associated w/smoking. "CIG-NO". (HSI)

➢ INTERPRETATION: Smokers showed lower peripheral levels of **omega-3**, when treated w/omega-3 fatty acids brought about a reduction in nicotine dependence. PubMed.

➢ **Milk thistle** damage protective; **Rhodiola, St John's wort, & fresh lime juice** helps for cessation.

➢ **Pycnogenol** - Smoker's Study Proves More Effective and Safer Than Aspirin. Greenmedinfo.com

Snoring

– causes range from lack of fitness/overweight, drinking alcohol before bed, smoking, & nasal congestion due to allergies. Food allergies may be an overlooked cause. Start w/AIP elimination diet

Stretch Marks – new chemical creams on market may work.

➤ **Fish oil capsules** inside/cocoa butter on the outside

Stress/Sleep

Adaptogens: ashwagandha, Rhodiola, Holy basil, cordyceps, Licorice root, Eleuthero, Astragalus, Maca, Schisandra….

➤ **Ashwagandha/Withania** – used in India for 3,000+ yrs to treat stress/chronic fatigue/improved memory/blood sugar/cortisol levels/anxiety/depression/sleep. 47 different beneficial compounds w/studies found it effective. (Stengler)

➤ **Rhodiola** (roseroot) – used for decades. 180+ studies published as improves short-term memory/concentration/alleviates stress-induced insomnia/ depression/poor appetite/irritability/hypertension/ headaches. (Dr Lark)

➤ **Schisandra** - staple of traditional medicine for centuries, known to help protect against adrenal fatigue/support healthy inflammation levels/fights free radicals/seeks out stress hormones & helps neutralize them. Organixx.com

➤ **Gotu Kola** – + good 4 agitation/anxiety/**insomnia**, epilepsy, hyperactivity (too much = rash + sedation)

➤ **Valarian root** – (nature's Valium-sleep) +**skullcap**+ **GABA** - increases brain serotonin, GABA calming effect. As effective as Serax w/o side effects. 300-500 mg 1 hr before bed. For children – 6-12 yrs = 160-320 mg VR + 80-160 mg **lemon balm** (German study) (Whitaker/Stengler)

➤ **Holy Basil or tulsa** – another highly studied adaptogens. It is antimicrobial, anti-diabetic, anti-inflammatory also helpful in the circulatory, immune, nervous systems & cancer treatments

➤ **Kava Kava** – Hawaiian root. Used for decades as stress/sleep drink. Not to be taken regularly/long term (over 30 days).

➤ **Essential oils** – lavender/doTerra serenity for stress/sleep.

> **Review diet** – no caffeine/sugar + add Ca/Mg/Zinc/ Potassium/Phosphorus + chamomile/peppermint tea. (Clark)

Thyroid/Hypothyroid

Auto-immune spectrum linked to gluten sensitivity, fluoride toxicity, chlorine, selenium/iodine deficiencies, leaky gut, parasites, SIBO, fungal overgrowth. **AIP dietary protocol** can decrease antibodies in as little as 21 days. See 'healing diets'

> **Siberian Ginseng**– or eleuthero. Extremely powerful stimulant properties that give the gland the energy it needs to function. Generally recommended dose is around 100 mg 2x/day before breakfast and before lunch.

> **Bacopa** – One study concluded that regular intake can reduce hypothyroidism symptoms < 41% w/no negative side-effects.

> **Ashwagandha** – adaptogen; Ayurvedic potent antioxidant directly affect thyroid. Studied to improve thyroid function & fight off free radicals; stress response.

> **Bladderwack** –This algae is an excellent source of iodine - "fuel" needed by the thyroid. It reduces the size of goiters usually associated with thyroid problems. Take as a preventive measure as stimulates production of thyroid.

> **Other support**: Boswellia, myrrh, ginger, flax & chia seeds, B12, D3, **selenium drops**, no fluoride, iodine rich foods - seaweed, kelp, radish, parsley, fish, seafood, eggs, bananas, cranberries, strawberries, Himalayan/pink crystal salt.

> **Gut support** - berberine, quercetin, bone broth collagen

Ulcers/Heartburn/Acid reflux/Diarrhea –

* **Ulcers** = maybe helicobacter pylori infection. 20% of Am/50% world have in stomach until aggravated by injury/meds (NSAIDs = 2nd leading cause) = blood test. Plain Yogurt w/lactobacillus+ Bifidobacterium can help reduce residual H pylori. (several)

* **Diarrhea** = many: 1). Clostridium difficile infection linked to Prilosec®, Prevacid®, Zantac®, NSAIDs use. 2). After anti-biotics. 3). Viral inf./bact'l toxins - food poisoning. 4). Traveler's = E coli. Most pass shortly. Eating banana's will slow

__Heartburn/acid reflux__ = may be **weak** HCl-pepsin. GERD linked to 1/3rd of esophageal cancer/44% ↑ risk of hip fracture/ ↑ stomach cancer risk. **Do digestion test.** "Purple pill" depletes bones by dropping Ca absorption by 41-61% - Am Jl Med.

➢ **If low levels of HCL/pepsin**. IV inj. until dig tests are normal. Then all oral. Zinc/selenium + essential minerals + Vit B_{12} & B-complex halts/reverses problem 70%.
  ✓ **Step 1**= dig. tested/dig. replacement therapy of betaine hydrochloride-pepsin or glutamic acid hydro-chloride-pepsin 1 cap./day (5,7 ½, or 10 grains) before meals 2-3 days. If no problems, 2 caps/day, continue to gradually ↑ to 40-90/meal. Need Dr monitoring (www. acam.org).
  ✓ **Step 2**= 30 mg **zinc** 2 x's/day; 4 mg **copper** diff. times than Zn; 1000 mg **taurine** between meals; 800 IU **Vit E;** 300 mcg **selenium**; 80 mg **bilberry** 2 x's/day. Expect sev. mos before any signs - needs to build up. (Dr J Wright)

➢ **Seabuckthorn** – seed oil caps/juice/creams/teas. Treat burns/grafts/infections/**gastric ulcers**/reduces inflamemation/ support liver/retard tumor growth/anti-bact'l (HSI)

➢ **Potters acidosis** – 2-3 tabs 3x/day after meals for several wks. www.herbal-direct.com or www.academyhealth.com

➢ **"Gasterol"** – a safe, natural blend of 5 organic herbs – Licorice root/L-glutamine/L-glycine/slippery elm bark/ Marshmallow root/Papaya/turmeric/fennel to strengthen/ rebuild stomach lining/aid digestion/gas/bloating. (HSI)

➢ **Heartburn** – start simple w/1 T *__raw apple cider vinegar__* before meals. Next, add digestive enzymes - root cause is too little acid. Next, eliminating carbonation/alcohol/coffee/non-herbal tea/chocolate/spicy foods. Add **Aloe Vera** 600 mg cap or 4 T extract 3x/day before meals. After 1 wk, add homeo "**Nux vomica**" 2 tabs 30C 2x/day until gone. (Dr Stengler) or **"Raphacholin"** – black radish + cholic acid + charcoal (can deactivate meds/not w/gallbladder issues). (HSI)

➢ **Peptic Ulcer** – **DGL** – 1 of most effective for this problem. Chew 2 caps at least 15 mins before each meal. (Stengler)

➢ **Pectin** – supp. taken at onset. May interfere w/meds.

➢ **Slippery Elm** - remedy for symptoms of chronic GI problems - leaky gut, ulcerative colitis, Crohn's disease, IBS

➢ **Zinc-carnosine** – 150 mg/day relieves symptoms/ kills infection/heals **ulcers**. Dissolves in stomach. Adheres to ulcer on lining & promotes mucus barrier. Prescription in Japan w/big improvement in 70% in 8 wks. (HSI)

➢ **Sulfur** – homeopathic = cellular detox brings energy back, detox's digestive tract (**ulcers/diarrhea/IBS**), relieves skin ailments (rashes/boils/psoriasis/eczema). Deficiency symptoms = always warm, sweats easily, no blankets, thirsty + likes sweet, spicy foods, fats, beer. Other applications = head-aches/insomnia/hot flashes/sore throat. 2 - 6C potency tabs 2/day for 2 weeks. For skin = may flare up temporarily due to detox. (Stengler)

➢ **Foods:** Garlic (5 gm/day), Grapefruits, probiotics, broccoli sprouts, manuka honey, mastic gum, marshmallow tea, ginger, baking soda, rosemary, aloe vera juice, raw organic apple cider vinegar (1 T in water).

➢ **Probiotics** – after antibiotics to restore nat'l intestinal bacterial flora w/probiotic capsules. (several sources)

Urinary infections/UTI's

➢ **Uva ursi** – herb works in 3 ways: releases hydro-quinone into urine to kill bacteria, diuretic to flush out infection, alkalizes urine. 500 mg 4X's/day. (Stengler)

➢ **"UroLogic"** – specifically designed 4 bladder tone/fcn = Crateva nurvala + Equisetum arvense. May enhance diuretic/BP meds. 2-3 months optimal effects. (HSI)

➢ **Candida overgrowth** – can be. If gets worse with antibiotics. **Grapefruit seed ext** – Strong anti-microbial. Or **Goldenseal/ Berberine** – plant alkaloids anti-microbial; **L-Glutamine –** fuels immune cells. Dr Osborne

➢ **D-Mannose** - powder form found in unsweetened cranberry juice –1 tsp every 2-3 hrs (from compound Pharm.)

➢ **Horseradish** – fresh prepared; glycoside sinigrin, a natural anti-microbial works better than anti-biotics of acute UTI. Dr Axe

> **Lactobacilli** (pills or yogurt) after antibiotics to restore natural flora + Vit C 1000 mg for 5 days.

> **Burdock** – eczema/acne/chronic UTI's. Detoxifier = supports liver, destroys blood bacterial/yeast, improves lymphatic system/digestion. Rich in minerals/phytonutrients/stim's metabolism/healing. 300-500 mg 2-3/day (Stengler)

Venous insufficiency/Varicose Vein -

swelling/itching/tingling/numbness/cramps/distended veins - may be due to liver problem – see liver. (Dr Null)

> **Butcher's broom extract** (ruscogenin) w/10% total saponins 20-40 mg 2/day+Vit C (monitor - may ↑ BP) (Dr. J Wright) may be combined w/horse chestnut

> **Sepia** – made from ink of cuttlefish. Treats hormone-related conditions = PMS/menopause/fibrocystic breast /low libido/ prostate enlargement/psoriasis/incontinence during meno-pause/uterine prolapse/vaginitis/**varicose veins**. (Stengler)

> **Horse chestnut seed extract** – German FDA recommendation/British review confirmed; 50 g 2x/day tab/gel www.totaldiscountvitamins.com

> **Gotu Kola** – increases blood flow through veins in the legs.

> **Pycnogenol** – Univ in Italy study = alleviates swelling/ edema for those w/diabetes & varicose veins. Can be taken w/Hi BP meds. (Dr Stengler)

> 200-600 mg **Mag** & 400-800 IU **Vit E**/day + ↑ **fiber**

> **Ginkgo Biloba** – terpene lactones - bioflavonoids/anti-oxidants prevent/treat Alzheimer's + strokes, cataracts/ macular degen./diabetic retinopathy, protects blood vessels, ↓ inflammation, **relieves varicose veins**, thins blood (↓ BP). 120-360 mg/day. Careful w/Coumadin/aspirin. (Dr Stengler)

> **Bromelain** – pineapple enzyme aids protein digestion (IBS), thins blood/breaks down clots/plaques/angina, anti-inflam. (arthritis), **varicose veins**, mucus thinning agent (CF or sinu-sitis), improves surgery recovery time. 2,000 MCU/1,000 mg or 1,200 GDU/ 1,000 mg split into 500 mg 3x/day. (Stengler)

➢ **Witch hazel** – rubbed on the area improves conditions by 10-25% for several hrs.

➢ **Prevent/slow** – **bilberry/hawthorn** extracts = bio-flavonoids found in dark-colored berries like blue-berries/blackberries + increase fiber. (Dr J White) + Omega's, zinc, vit C, folate, glycine, collagen. May also be linked to hormone dysregulation. (Paleo mom)

Warts

❖ **Tea tree oil** (Melaleuca alternifora oil) = anti-inflam./analgesic/antiseptic/anti-bact'l/fungal/viral for acne/ athlete's foot/cold sores/cuts/insect bites/rashes/ **warts**/etc. 5% extract cream or gel, as soap, or 10 drops - 1 ts in water (not undiluted). Not for infants. (Stengler)

Weight loss weight problems are not always due to poor

diet/eating habits. Excessive weight is on the auto-immune spectrum & toxicity from pesticides/heavy metals. Need to *go organic*. Other things - from food **sensitivities/allergies** (see allergies) to **vit/min** imbalances (no drugs & only some sweeteners are safe - see diabetes) to **hormone** imbalances/adrenal fatigue/gut dysbiosis.

Start w/slow elimination diet removing 1 thing at a time for a week & continue. Starting with gluten (wheat/rye/barley/oats/corn) + all packaged/process, preservatives/MSG/etc.). After a week, cow dairy. Your goal may be dairy-free *ketogenic* (see 'healing diets').

➢ **Adrenal fatigue** – in-office physical testing or others. Many well-tested natural adrenal supp available to allow adrenals to "rest". Need Dr support. (Williams)

➢ **Hypothyroid** (TSH 2.0+)– **Bladderwack** + **L-tyrosine** provides thyroid support by Gaia Herbs. L-tyrosine + iodine + thyroid glandular = Solaray (Stengler)

➢ **Enzyme therapy** – many wt problems revolve around low stomach acid/improper digestion/nutrient absorption/liver issue (see liver). Good digestive enzyme containing bromelain/protease/lipase/amylase (= pancreatin 4X), betaine HCl/ox bile taken at every meal. (Stengler)

➢ **Tsao mi** – botanical Chinese plant in Duke Univ study to shed large amounts of weight for little cost. (Balch/Stengler)

➢ **Dehydroepiandrosterone** – (DHEA) Cuts insulin resistance/ burns fat; naturally diminishes w/age. Get tested. < 50 mg/day monitored by physician. (Stengler)

➢ **Cordyceps sinensis** Cs-4 extract – 2,400 mg of medicinal mushroom helps support DHEA production. (Stengler)

➢ **Cortisol – Ashwagandha** Sensoril (adaptogen) – reduces cortisol/helps deal w/stress/stress-related appetite/wt gain, fights fatigue, ↑ memory/sexual performance. (Stengler)

➢ **Gymnema Sylvestre** – staves off sugar cravings/ balances blood sugar. In test subjects, ↑ in # of insulin secreting beta cells – repair/regenerate new cells, ↑ activity of enzymes responsible for glucose uptake/ utilization. Researchers found in 1 control study w/ **Type I diabetes**, insulin requirement fell dramatically. **Type 2** study found ↑ insulin/reduced med's. 24-25% gymnemic acids 400-600 mg/day. (Stengler/Fuchs/HSI)

➢ **MCT oil** – natural; may actually empty fat cells/not store it. Current studies show ↓ food intake, ↑ energy expenditure/ endurance, anti-microbial (fungus). Replaces butter, veg. oil, make salad dressing, cooking/sautéing. Must be kept <325 °F.

➢ **Terrain Management** – studies reveal that microbiome of overweight patients differs from those of normal weight. They recommend 16+ strain **probiotics + fermented foods**.

➢ **"*Pain & Brain Rescue formula*"** – curcuminoids (**turmeric)** + Boswellia (anti-inflam.)= ↓ arthritis/neutralizes metabolic wastes, **Gugulipid** converts excess cholesterol/burns stored fat/↑ levels of prostacyclin to zap abnormal platelets/detox all major organs/ immune enhancer/anti-bact'l/viral/fungal, ↓ stress/fatigue, **Bioerine** to absorb/use nutrients,… Institute for Vibrant Living

➢ **Konjac mannan extract** – lowers BP & cholesterol + ***blocks fat absorption*** (careful – need fat to burn fat!)

- ➢ **Hoodia gordonii extract -** 500 mg (20:1) S. Africa – natural **appetite suppressant,** ↓ depression/anxiety/**sugar cravings** - no ephedra, caffeine. Beware of Mexican/So. Amer. knock-offs. Silver Edge Hlt/Nut GMP lab processed or Nature's Ben (HSI)

- ➢ **Fucoxanthin** – Carotenoid from brown seaweed ext - anti-oxidant & helps burn fat/increase metabolic rate. "*Biothin*" = Fucoxanthin +Hoodia +Irvengia. (Mercola.com)

- ➢ **L-Carnitine** – an amino acid shown to help convert body fat into energy + improve heart health + increases effectiveness of anti-oxidants Vit C & E (Dr Yale +)

- ➢ **LGB** – new Univ study = dramatically corrects the way body metabolizes food – permanently even total reversal of disease even for morbidly obese. (Dr Whitaker)

- ➢ **Arjuna** – well-proven cure for lowering LDL/overall chol-esterol/angina attacks w/o side effects (out performed ISMN) + ↓ systolic BP, ↓ **body mass index** (wt. loss), correct athero-sclerosis, fight several cancers & several bacterial infections. *Arjuna-Cardiac Tonic* (Himalaya USA 800-869-4640)

- ➢ **PYY** – London's Imperial College study = natural protein secreted in intestine - tells brain you're full helping to **reduce food intake** by 30-40%. (Whitaker)

- ➢ **Tamarind extract** – 8 wk placebo study found tames **appetite**, reduces cholesterol/triglycerides/BP/& subjects ate 15-30% less food. (Prev/Natural Fat-Loss Pharmacy)

- ➢ **Caralluma fimbriata** (Slimaluma) – listed as a veg & "famine food" in Indian Health Ministry's medicinal plants. Curbs appetite & reduces abdominal fat. 2 double-blind placebo trials w/500 mg taken 30-60 mins before breakfast/ dinner. 2nd study @ Western Geriatric RI in LA. (Stengler)

- ➢ **Chromium/cinnamon/ALA** – balance blood sugar/insulin levels & increase muscle/metabolism.

- ➢ **Phydrox** = green tea, chromium, hydroxycitric acid, glucomannan (www.phydrox.com)

➢ **Luo Han Guo** – see nat'l sweeteners in diabetes section.

➢ **Banaba plant** – lowers blood sugar by 32% in 3 wks for mild-mod **Type II** + lose weight. Active ingredient = corosolic acid. *"Glucosol/Normalose"* 48 mg/day. Harmony Co. (HSI)

➢ **Calcium/Magnesium** connection – 1000 mg each balances pH/cleans blood. Add Chlorophyll/minerals lacking = pH distress (norm 7.4) + helps ↓ belly fat. (sev sources)

➢ **Arginine & liquid potassium** – stimulates natural HGH production (injection too risky)

➢ **Irvingia gabonesis ext** – West African herb. Studies show supports optimal leptin sensitivity that signals fullness. In study, 150 mg 2x'/day, group lost 28 lbs/10 wks + reduced C-reactive protein levels & increased circulating adiponectin. (Mercola.com -**BioThin** = Irvingia +fucoxanthin + Hoodia).

➢ **Garcinia cambogia** – hydroxycycitrase (HCA) regulates appetite/maximizes carb. utilization/jump-starts metabolism/ burns fat/maintains cholesterol/triglyceride levels. Weight Guard Plus (NorthStar Nut)

➢ **Di-indole methane (DIM)** – a plant nutrient in cruciferous veggies that balances hormones/prevents estrogen dominance (menopausal/prostate problems)/fights depression/anxiety/ fatigue/hair loss/thyroid problems/reduces risk for abnormal cell growth. (Jl of Endocrine & Metabolism/Jl of Bio Chem/Br Jl of Cancer/Jl of Clinical Endocrinology) - + 600 mg **ALA** + 20 mg **vanadium** + Vit **E** + **magnesium** 250 mg + 1 t/day **flax seed.** (Dr Susan M Lark)

➢ **CLA -** omega-3 missing from food supply that promotes weight loss. Found in *grazing* beef products. (several sources)

➢ **Gurmar** – Ayurvedic herb slows sugar absorption/con-version to body fat + suppresses sweet cravings (Weil)

➢ **Flaxseed meal/oil** = omega-3 fatty acids. 1T 2x/day oil or sprinkle on food or 1000 mg. (many sources)

➢ **Apple-cider Vinegar** – see multi-symptomatic.

➤ **Probiotic Lactobacillus gasseri** - study subjects averaged 4.6% decrease in abdominal fat+3.3% decrease in subcutaneous fat over 12 wk study. (Mercola)

➤ **Garcinia cambogia** – hydroxycycitrase (HCA) regulates appetite/maximizes carb. utilization/jump-starts metabolism/ burns fat/maintains cholesterol/triglyceride levels. Weight Guard Plus (NorthStar Nut)

➤ **"Artic weed"** eat or steep in tea – ↑ brain serotonin levels by 30% to ↓ depression symptoms/provides energy boost/loose wt. Russian studies since 70's. (Inglis)

➤ **Fiber (60 gm/day)**– on any diet, don't get enough. Studies adding fiber only is showing wt loss! Benefiber added to anything - even water (dissolves clear w/no taste) or sprinkle **flaxseed meal** on food. Avocadoes = 12 g, raspberries & blackberries = 8 g, acorn squash = 6 g, black beans = 8 g, sweet potato = 5 g. (several)

➤ **Food – many sources** (use "glycemic index")
  ✓ **All fats** are not created equal. Omega 3s & mono-unsaturated are best (fish/flax/nuts/seeds/olive oils (EVOO)/coconut/MCT/avocados/black cumin seed oil. Bad fats = highly processed/poly-unsaturated/ trans-fats/hydrogenated/ … no GMO/corn/safflower/ vegetable/soybean/canola/margarines/packaged baked goods.
  ✓ **Eat good carbs** = low sugar fruits/veggies – berries, squash, apples, lemons, sweet potatoes, cucumbers, celery, onions, bell peppers, roots,…. Grapefruit – ½ before each meal (Scripps Clinic San Diego) helps regulate insulin levels.
  ✓ **Good protein** = organic meat (grass fed or wild caught are best) - fish, chicken, beef, lamb, nuts, seeds, bone broth protein,….
  ✓ **Herbal Tea** – drinking warm lemon (fresh) water in the morning with raw apple cider vinegar stimulates digestion, immune system, balances pH,.. add some *match green tea* powder & honey or stevia for great wake up drink.

- Exercise – most consider walking the best. Fat burning level is slower & longer = stroll for 30 mins & work up to 1 hr. Some (Dr Hyman) suggest intervals of higher, short-bursts for 30-60 sec during walk – up/down stairs, high knees, skipping, jumping jacks,… 4x in your hour walk.

- **Fat Flush Plan book** by Ann Louise Gittleman. Sound diet w/nutrition. Basically, no wheat (70% of pop sensitive), no dairy, no processed foods + Flaxseed oil/meal & cranberry juice (unsweetened).

- **Eat Fat, Get Thin** book – Dr Mark Hyman

Wrinkles

- **Antioxidant creams** = 10% Vit C cream/solution + CoQ_{10}, ALA, & DMAE from a compounding pharmacist or Rejuvenating Skin Cream 800-985-8065/www.ucprx.com. (Dr Stengler +)

- **Ubiquinone** – converted CoQ 10 enzyme that ↓ w/age = deterioration tied to heart/baldness/wrinkles/eyesight/ hearing/gums/arthritis/age spots/bladder control/& prostate. Noble prize winner Dr P Mitchell, Dr Wm V Judy, AMA, JIM, JN, US Gov NIH, UCLA Med School, Indiana Univ med school. "*Ubitol*" – BioNutrigenics, 800-206-9872)/ "*Cardigen*" – Swiss labs, 800-301-9471)

- **Tamanu oil/Calophyllum inophyllum** – effective cicatrizing agent w/anti-bact'l/infam & antioxidant prop's. Calophyllic acid is unique fatty acid here + xanthones + coumarins. Used topically for eczema/ psoriasis/shingles/ rheumatism/neuralgia = 100% solution. Wounds/blemishes/ wrinkles = 50/50 solution (HSI)

- **Others**: collagen powder, Vit C skin serum, ceramides, Hyaluronic acid, germanium essential oil.

Tid-Bits

Our food supply is dropping in nutritional value due to a decrease in our soil's mineral content + decrease in Omega-3 & -6 due to our grain-fed cows & chickens instead of free-ranging it (not just cage-free/grass fed). The antibiotics & hormones they feed our livestock may be responsible for decreasing our immune systems & increasing resistance/mutations in bacteria/viruses.

Genetically modified/engineered food (GMO) – by definition = any crops where new DNA sections are added from another plant/bacteria to increase food production or to make other products – mainly corn/soy/rice/cotton/sugar beets/rapeseed (canola).

Recently, some US areas have opted for "no GMO's" where food crops grow as many of these GMO's are altered to produce pharmaceuticals, plastics, detergents, pesticides, etc. These GMO crop's pollen can cross-pollinate into our food crops. "The use of food crops for this purpose threatens the safety of our entire food supply", per Karen Perry Stillerman, senior analyst for UCS. "In 2002, 1 company allowed corn containing a pig vaccine to mix with 1000's of bushels of soybeans in a Nebraska grain elevator. And Pharma-corn may have cross-pollinated with feed corn in Iowa. In 2006, an unapproved GMO rice contaminated domestic and export consumer rice… Due to regulatory oversights, …these events suggest contamination is inevitable under current conditions".

As for the food-producing GMO's, 60+ % of our processed foods now contain hidden GMO's. Currently, an increasing # of experts suspect they are responsible for huge jump in food allergies, microbiome dysbiosis, sugar dysregulation, mutated amino acid structures, & now the cancer issues with ***glyphosate on a cumulative basis***. Per Jeffery M Smith, director of Institute of Responsible Technology, the side effects from animal testing include: stunted growth/impaired immune systems/reduced digestive enzymes/bleeding stomachs/abnormal to pre-cancerous intestinal cells/impaired blood cell development/mis-shapened liver, pancreas, testicular cell structures/altered gene expression/enlarged livers, pancreas, intestines/inflamed kidneys & lung tissue/liver & kidney lesions/high blood sugar-insulin regulation/fertility problems, etc. In the early 1990s, scientific consensus at FDA was that GMOs were dangerous & was ordered to promote it anyway.

Many countries have declined our "free seed gifts" opting not to be "guinea pigs" in what has been dubbed the biggest human experiment in history.

Prolotherapy – a treatment/permanent cure for pain, arthritis, inflam. Dr. injects irritant solution that triggers healing response that strengthens ligaments/tendons by 40%. Currently only 300 Dr's in US but many in other countries (Bottomline Health)

Plastic – Our oil dependence is killing us. PCB/BPA are oil-derived products. Water bottle testing is showing BPA leaching from the plastic into the water we buy + microparticles in the water as well. Biggest release occurs from freezing/ heating food/liquids (baby formula) as **toxic** molecules from the plastic are absorb into the food/liquid. American Association for Cancer Research now states plastic may be contributing to breast cancer. Dr Stengler recommends checking the recycling code on the bottom of the container. '7' is no, '5' is better. Better off using glass, steel, or ceramic. Also, beware of children's baby bottles (more leaching w/every wash) & plastic toys they put in their mouths as saliva breaks it down.

They can make biodegradable plastics. Some water bottle companies have tried it on the market but these bottles cost several pennies more & people go cheap keeping this technology from taking off. So, vote for change w/purchases!

Bug Bites - DEET can impair cell function in parts of your brain - rats in the lab = death & behavioral changes with frequent or prolonged DEET use. Plus, it can combine w/other skin products & meds to cause further problems. Cinnamon oil performed better than DEET. Natural insect repellant with a combo's of citronella, lemongrass oil, peppermint oil, & vanillin. After – use aloe vera/ Calendula/ Chamomile/Cinnamon/Cucumbers/Honey/Lavender oil/Neem Oil/Tea Tree Oil/toothpaste. (Mercola)

Wheat/Gluten sensitivity/Celiac disease – Studies show 250 known symptoms. Per Gittleman (HSI), 40-**70%** of population is sensitive & most have no real symptoms. Other sources document 1 in 266 people worldwide & 1 in 133 in US (twice as many) have celiac disease. Per NIH, that is about 3 million Americans. The rates for sensitivity are much higher. The problem with wheat/rye/

barley/oats/corn is their glutens are resistant to our protein digestive enzymes. In some, this problem becomes an ***autoimmune response*** (not just Celiac Disease). Symptoms range from bloating to fatigue, depression to infertility, or misdiagnosed for years as IBS, Lupus, diabetes, CF, malnutrition, mineral deficiencies, osteoporosis, and so on.

The term you may be more familiar with is *"**leaky gut syndrome**"* as particles of gluten pass through the intestinal barrier and your immune system recognizes it as a foreign object and reacts (immune response) in ALL HUMANS. Gluten is like sandpaper to our intestines leading to holes torn in the intestinal walls so that intestinal contents leaks into the blood stream setting off even more immune response that can end up in your joint, your thyroid, our brain,…no organs/tissues are immune to these effects.

Why go gluten free? You probably have a sensitivity to it & don't know it. It is actually easier than you think. More people are becoming aware so more and more foods are becoming available. First step, you need to stop all processed foods – no more "prepared" dishes/foods from stores. Restaurants are now offering gluten-free items. Second step, touch up your home cooking recipes. Chick pea pasta, almond/coconut flour breads, muffins, pancake/ baking mixes, etc. are all available. Health food stores are full of them and they are starting to make their way into mainstream grocery stores. Do be careful of store products if blood sugar issues as rice flour spikes insulin even more than wheat.

EMF – the research is getting stronger & stronger even though the signal is too. EMF messes with calcium channels & insulin in the body wreaking havoc. Start the process of lowing your exposure: turn off wifi at night, cell phone on airplane mode during sleep, other protection-lowering devises are available.

FSM (frequency specific micro-current) – FDA banned years ago considered by some to be a bureaucratic corruption conspiracy is now legal. Research shows it increases protein synthesis rates to help re-build damaged tissue. Now, 100s of Dr's now trained to use for chronic diseases - macular degeneration, heart disease, fibromyalgia, hyperthyroidism, carpal tunnel syndrome, diabetes, etc. (Rowen MD)

About the Author

Present: I can tell you, "Food is Medicine"! As of 2014, I had over 15 auto-immune spectrum conditions/symptoms (asthma/allergies/arthritis/edema/eczema/candida overgrowth/mild hypothyroidism/leaky gut/diabetes/obesity/stage 3+ kidney disease/NAFLD/regrown cartilage for bone-on-bone knees/brain fog/anxiety/panic attacks/40 yrs of pain,...) taking all kinds of supplements & still going downhill not recognizing my root cause was food. I was trained in the 'old' failed food pyramid with high grains & low fat.

I have walked the walk. When I change my diet, everything changed – it took about 1 year to losing 90 lbs (kept it off for 3 yrs), 2 more years to reverse it all by going gluten-free, dairy free, grain free, organic, low carb, high fat, & detoxing. I now am healthier than I have been in 40+ yrs & have more energy than I can ever remember having. This is all possible. The body can heal.

The Beginning: I was born & raised in So. Cal. I became aware of alternatives when I was 11 years old. I was already an accomplished athlete. In about 1 year, I grew 6 inches & was 'told' my bone & muscle structures had gone astray causing severe pain in my feet, knees, & back. I was diagnosed with ***arthritis.*** The regular medical community abandoned me as incurable & surgery, pills, and pain were to be my life & an end to my athletics. Add on top of this in same year, ***allergies & asthma.***

My grandmother stepped in & started my path to recovery with alternative treatments. I responded very quickly to orthotics & chiropractic work. By the time I graduated from high school, I had a 12 yrs old world record, several national age-group titles, traveled around the world competing in track & field. When athletic scholarship offers started coming my way, I decided to major in Biology. I had a good run in track & field through college (1 national champ/4 x All –Am/10 top-10 rankings & 2 Olympic trials). I did change my major several times from Biology to Kinesiology to Public Health increase the span of my knowledge until I decided I wanted a career as a Sports Medicine Dietician to bring my knowledge of nutrition together with my love for high-performance sports. I did my senior thesis on "Mineral Losses in Sweat & How They affect Body Balance".

Although I received my BS in Nutrition/Food Science from California State Polytechnic University @ Pomona, CA, I was unable to pursue my career choice as the path to professional sports had dried up & financially unable to pursue further into dietetics to become 'registered' Dietitian. I still remained hungry to furthering my knowledge, especially in natural cures, which were not part of that curriculum.

I did not further that pursuit until many years later when my father, who, in my youth, was a big, strong, athletic man, became ill with diabetes, heart disease, a stroke, & later Parkinson's & started taking huge numbers of prescription medications & drinking huge amounts of diet soda. I watched him deteriorate year after year as he was prescribed more and more medications that seemed to just accelerate the declination of his health.

I tried to intervene but my father, being old school medicine where doctors know everything, he was not willing to step on his doctor's toes as they must know more than me. I then, tried to talk to his doctor's and found they had no knowledge of any toxic affects of diet foods nor any of the alternatives I thought might help him. I explained to these Doc's that unless they discussed these options with him, he would not try them. I recommended to my father to seek a naturopathic doctor and he believed he was getting the best care available with conventional medicine.

I accelerated my research in his final years continuing to try to help him. In doing so, I discovered there was so much information about so many different ailments that I started making a list from books, subscriptions, newsletters, peer-reviewed articles, e-zines, clinical studies, research institutes like Harvard, etc. This book is the result of all that accumulation. At first, I did not record where information came from but as time went on and I decided to share this information, I started adding the sources of the information. Hence, some listings do not have original source and others do to allow readers the opportunity to investigate and read the information for themselves.

After my own experience, I have become well versed in dietary protocols, leaky gut, terrain management, obtained my Gastro-Intestinal Mastery certification from the Integrative Medicine Academy & now coach others to do use food as medicine as I did.

I have now also explored radiation damage (EMF), bioenergetics, and psychosomatic disorders in my quest for better health for myself. I am now healthier and happier with myself than I have been in 50 years. May we all strive to reach a higher sense of body and mind health.